Collagen Biomaterials

Edited by Nirmal Mazumder
and Sanjiban Chakrabarty

Published in London, United Kingdom

Collagen Biomaterials
http://dx.doi.org/10.5772/intechopen.95635
Edited by Nirmal Mazumder and Sanjiban Chakrabarty

Contributors
Nirmal Mazumder, Kausalya Neelavara Makkithaya, Sharmila Nadumane, Guan-Yu Zhuo, Sanjiban Chakrabarty, Dar-Jen Hsieh, Periasamy Srinivasan, Bruno Silvestrini, Matteo Innocenti, Chuen Yan Cheng, Amit Kumar Verma, Shunji Yunoki, Eiji Kondo, Kazunori Yasuda, Lajos Csönge, Ágnes Bozsik, Zoltán Tóth Bagi, Róbert Gyuris, Dóra K. Csönge, János Kónya, Sougata Ghosh, Bishwarup Sarkar, Ratnakar Mishra, Nanasaheb Thorat, Sirikanjana Thongmee

First published in London, United Kingdom, 2022 by IntechOpen
IntechOpen is the global imprint of INTECHOPEN LIMITED, registered in England and Wales, registration number: 11086078, 5 Princes Gate Court, London, SW7 2QJ, United Kingdom

British Library Cataloguing-in-Publication Data
A catalogue record for this book is available from the British Library

Additional hard and PDF copies can be obtained from orders@intechopen.com

Collagen Biomaterials
Edited by Nirmal Mazumder and Sanjiban Chakrabarty
p. cm.
Print ISBN 978-1-80355-411-2
Online ISBN 978-1-80355-412-9
eBook (PDF) ISBN 978-1-80355-413-6

Meet the editor

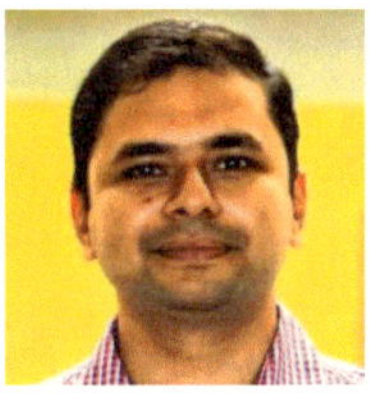

Dr. Nirmal Mazumder is an assistant professor in the Department of Biophysics, Manipal School of Life Sciences, Manipal Academy of Higher Education, India. He obtained his Ph.D. from National Yang Ming Chiao Tung University, Taipei, Taiwan in 2013. From 2013 to 2016, he worked as a postdoctoral fellow at the University of Virginia, USA, and the Italian Institute of Technology, Genoa, Italy. He has been developing nonlinear optical microscopes, including two-photon fluorescence, second harmonic generation, and coherent anti-Stokes Raman scattering for biomedical applications. He has published several research articles in peer-reviewed international journals, books, and book chapters. He serves as a reviewer and guest editor for prestigious journals and member of national and international scientific societies and organizations.

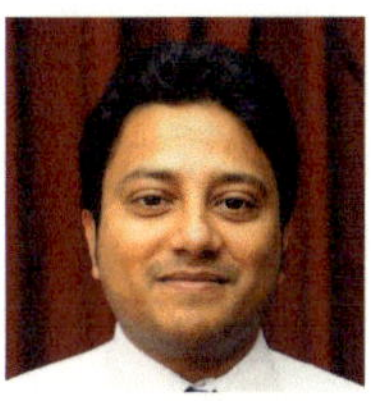

Dr. Sanjiban Chakrabarty is an assistant professor and coordinator, at the Center for DNA Repair and Genome Stability, Department of Cell and Molecular Biology, Manipal School of Life Sciences, Manipal Academy of Higher Education (MAHE), India. Trained in biochemistry, he obtained his Ph.D. in Human Genetics from MAHE in 2013. He worked as a postdoctoral fellow at the Erasmus University Medical Center, Rotterdam, the Netherlands. His research interests and expertise are in cancer genomics, mitochondrial biology, and DNA damage response. He is a member of several national and international scientific societies and an external Ph.D. expert committee member. He has published several research articles in international journals and has two patents in his name. He serves as a reviewer and guest editor for many prestigious journals.

Contents

Preface **IX**

Section 1
Health **1**

Chapter 1 **3**
Collagen Involvement in Health, Disease, and Medicine
by Bruno Silvestrini, Chuen Yan Cheng and Matteo Innocenti

Chapter 2 **15**
Supercritical Carbon Dioxide Facilitated Collagen Scaffold Production for Tissue Engineering
by Periasamy Srinivasan and Dar-Jen Hsieh

Chapter 3 **37**
Nanoparticle Based Collagen Biomaterials for Wound Healing
by Kausalya Neelavara Makkithaya, Sharmila Nadumane, Guan-Yu Zhuo, Sanjiban Chakrabarty and Nirmal Mazumder

Chapter 4 **57**
Thermal Manipulation of Human Bone Collagen Membrane (SoftBone) and Platelet-Rich Fibrin (PRF) Membranes
by Lajos Csönge, Ágnes Bozsik, Zoltán T. Bagi, Róbert Gyuris, Dóra K. Csönge and János Kónya

Section 2
Tissue Engineering **73**

Chapter 5 **75**
Collagen-Based Biomaterial as Drug Delivery Module
by Amit Kumar Verma

Chapter 6 **115**
Collagen Based 3D Printed Scaffolds for Tissue Engineering
by Sougata Ghosh, Bishwarup Sarkar, Ratnakar Mishra, Nanasaheb Thorat and Sirikanjana Thongmee

Chapter 7 **133**
Mechanical Methods of Producing Biomaterials with Aligned Collagen Fibrils
by Shunji Yunoki, Eiji Kondo and Kazunori Yasuda

Preface

Collagen is a ubiquitous protein, present in most tissues and a major contributor to their underlying architecture. Recent advances in molecular and structural biology have contributed to a better understanding of the structure and function of collagen. Collagen biomaterial is frequently employed for various applications such as a medium for delivery of drugs and genes, scaffold to support the growth of tissues, and much more. *Collagen Biomaterials* highlights some of the remarkable properties of collagen that make it one of the most widely studied and used biomaterials. With the advent of tissue engineering techniques, there has been a significant increase in the research interest in the development of novel applications of collagen as a biomaterial. The preference for collagen as biomaterials is also fueled by the fact that it is readily accessible, biocompatible with the human body, extremely malleable to one's requirements, and more importantly, biodegradable. Translational research on the various applications of collagen as a biomaterial is extremely important due to the diversity of roles that collagen and its various molecular types play in the body. Collagen is a major component of the extracellular matrix (ECM) of tissues and contributes to the stability, support, and growth of the tissue. Although there have been numerous books on collagen describing its structure, synthesis, and other properties, there have been only a few books that discuss collagen as a biomaterial. The current volume elucidates the various applications collagen biomaterials have found in the fields of medicine and tissue engineering.

Collagen Biomaterials is a collection of chapters that explore the various aspects of collagen that make it desirable as a biomaterial scaffold, its various applications, and the scope for further research. Chapter 1 by Silvestrini et al. discusses the involvement of collagen in health, disease, and medicine. The chapter elucidates the role of collagen in many functions of the body. The authors discuss the metabolism of collagen, factors affecting it, the disorders related to collagen deficiency, and its impact on the general health of individuals. Chapter 2 by Periasamy Srinivasan and Dar-Jen Hsieh discusses and compares the role of supercritical carbon dioxide extraction technology in the production of collagen scaffold biomaterials from various tissues and organs with the traditional decellularization techniques used in the production of collagen biomaterials, in the field of tissue engineering, and its implication in the field of regenerative medicine. The authors also elucidate the physicochemical properties, toxicity, biocompatibility, and bioactivity both in vitro and in vivo of the collagen scaffolds that are produced using carbon dioxide extraction technology. Chapter 3 by Makkithaya et al. discusses the application of collagen biomaterials for wound healing. The authors also elucidate the production of collagen in amalgamation with nanoparticles and its advantages for wound healing. The chapter also briefly describes the various applications of nano collagen in the biomedical field for wound healing. Chapter 4 by Bozsik et al. analyzes the various features of freeze-dried human collagen membranes consisting of cortical bone (SoftBone=SB) and folded platelet-rich fibrin (F-PRF) membranes after thermal modification and freeze-drying. The authors also compare the resistance properties shown by collagen and PRF membranes. Detailed knowledge of the properties of collagen and PRF membranes is important during guided bone regeneration surgeries in dentistry. Chapter 5 by Amit Kumar Verma discusses the various methods of crosslinking collagen polymers and their implications in the field of pharmacology. The chapter also discusses the various formulations of collagen biomaterials that are used as a vehicle for the delivery of drugs. Chapter 6 by Ghosh et al. elucidates the application of 3D printing technologies to create collagen scaffolds. The authors discuss the various ways in which collagen in combination with other materials such as oxidized hyaluronic acid, bioinks, heparin sulfate, and many others can be used as scaffolds and implants in tissue engineering and regenerative medicine. The development of biomaterials with collagen as a structural protein is known to be beneficial in terms of the bioactivity and biocompatibility of said biomaterial because collagen is the structural component in the ECM of most tissues in the human body. Chapter 7 by Yunoki et al. elucidates the various mechanical methods employed for the fabrication of such biomaterials in considerable detail. The authors also summarize other well-known methods for producing collagen biomaterials.

The authors' contributions to this book as well as their timely responses to the reviewers' comments are greatly appreciated. We appreciate the reviewers for investing their time to make constructive suggestions and recommendations on the chapters, which helped us to improve the quality of content in the book. We also acknowledge the support and suggestions received from our colleagues. Our special thanks to Josip Knapić at IntechOpen for his contributions to the book. Most importantly, we wish our readers a pleasant and productive reading experience.

Nirmal Mazumder
Department of Biophysics,
Manipal School of Life Sciences,
Manipal Academy of Higher Education,
Manipal, Karnataka, India

Sanjiban Chakrabarty
Department of Cell and Molecular Biology,
Manipal School of Life Sciences,
Manipal Academy of Higher Education,
Manipal, Karnataka, India

Section 1

Health

Chapter 1

Collagen Involvement in Health, Disease, and Medicine

Bruno Silvestrini, Chuen Yan Cheng and Matteo Innocenti

Abstract

This chapter discusses the physiologic, metabolic, and clinical aspects of collagen, including the role of nutritional factors in a new nosographic entity, called "extended collagen carential disease." Except water and possibly fats, carbohydrates, and other structural proteins, perhaps there is more collagen in the mammalian body than anything else. Moreover, collagen participates in almost all of the body functions, adjusting its structure constantly in response to changes in environment, development, growth, and external clues. Collagens found in bones and nails are different from collagens found in body fluids and other biological structures, such as basement membrane, skin, tendons, muscles, and hair. The ubiquity of collagen functions accounts for its phylogenetic ubiquity, involving any tissue, organ, and apparatus. This is shown by the so-called "collagen carential disease," involving nails, hair, osteoarticular and gastrointestinal systems. For instance, the Ehlers-Danlos syndrome describes another group of genetic collagen disorders, affecting the collagen processing and structure. Some of them are inherited in an autosomal dominant manner, while others emerge in the absence of essential nutritional factors. It is the case of Vitamin C, which plays a critical role in the maintenance of a normal mature collagen network. Hence, the idea of an "extended collagen carential disease," applicable to the absence of essential nutritional factors.

Keywords: collagen physiology, collagen pathology, collagen medicine, collagen physiopathology, collagen supplement

1. Introduction

The term collagen designates a family of proteins, which spread throughout the whole organism, linking its parts and carrying out a precise physiological role. In contrast to spherical globular, collagen is composed of linear, fiber-like structures. All cells and tissues are supported by a network of collagen fibers, the arrangement of which appears to be specifically site adaptive [1]. Its structural domain, namely tropocollagen, is a molecule of about 300 kDa, 300 nm long, and 1.5 nm in diameter and mainly composed of glycine (Gly) lysine (Lys) and proline (Pro).

The hydroxylation of Pro and Lys is catalyzed by prolyl 3-hydroxylase, prolyl 4-hydroxylase and lysil-hydroxylase, and these reactions all require free O_2, ferrous iron, α-ketoglutarate, and ascorbic acid. Prolyl-hydroxylase hydroxylates the third carbon, whereas prolyl 4-hydroxilase hydroxylates the fourth carbon in the proline ring. An adequate amount of 4-hydroxyproline helps to stabilize the triple helix of collagen in the human body. Therefore, when its content is not enough, the newly synthetized collagen is denatured. It is the case of scurvy and local tissue hypoxia [2, 3]. This process increases the possibilities of hydrogen bonds, decreasing the steric hindrance of the molecule and improving its resistance to decay and disintegration.

In addition to the high content of Gly, Lys, and Pro, a distinctive feature of tropocollagen is the so-called α-chains, consisting of amino acid repeats of (Gly-X-Y)n, where X and Y are typically proline (Pro) or hydroxylated proline, 3-hydroxyproline or 4-hydroxyproline.

Like other proteins, collagen has primary, secondary, tertiary structural elements. It has also a quaternary structure similar to other complex oligomeric proteins, which are characterized by having multiple polypeptide chains or subunit [4]. To date, some XXVIII different types of collagens have been identified.

About 44 genes, which typically have the "COL" prefix, are associated with the biosynthesis of collagen, which begins with turning on genes, which are associated with the formation of an α peptide. Following the transcription into the collagen mRNA, it enters into the cytoplasm, where a translational process begins. Once the synthesis of the new peptide is finished, it goes into the rough end plasmatic reticulum (rER) for posttranslational process, forming a pre-pro-collagen. Removal of the signal peptide on the N-terminal and the glycosylation occur to transform the pre-pro-collagen into the procollagen, which is packaged into vesicle destined to Golgi apparatus. Herein, procollagen undergoes last posttranslational modification, representing by oligosaccharides addition, before being secreted out of the cell, wherein the action of collagen peptidase serves to obtain the formation of tropocollagen. Outside the cell, lysin oxidase acts on the amino acids lysines and hydroxylysines producing aldehyde groups, for covalent binding between tropocollagen polymer, forming the so-called collagen fibril.

Type I, II, III, and IV collagens are the most abundant collagens found in several tissues.

Type I collagen is a fibrillar-type collagen and the most abundant in the composition of several tissues. It forms connective tissues, tendons, skin, artery walls, cornea, fibrocartilage, and the organic matrix of bone and teeth, serving to the deposit of the mineral matrix, conferring further stiffness and hardness to these tissues. Without its action, calcium salts would go unused. Type I collagen mutations occur in several genetic diseases, such as osteogenesis imperfecta and Ehlers-Danlos syndrome (EDS). In the adult, type II collagen, instead, is the major structural component of the hyaline cartilage, vitreous humor of the eye, and it is also found in other tissues, such as the nucleus pulposus of the intervertebral disc, whereas type III is the structural component in hollow organs, such as intestines and uterus. Lastly, type IV collagen is a type of collagen found primarily in the skin within the basement membrane zone and also the testis. It also forms basal lamina, eye lens, and also serves as part of the filtration system in capillaries and the glomeruli of nephron in the kidney. In essence, the tropocollagen represents a common matrix and the unifying element of the variegated collagen family.

Collagen has two fundamental biological properties: a mechanistic effect, of support and protection, and a trophic one. The first is comparable to the function of cement that composes and covers a building, supporting and protecting it from foreign elements. The mechanistic action is so strong to be used in the protection of marble monuments from acid rain [3]. A new in vitro test has been recently developed to measure the barrier effect of collagen against the erosive action of hydrochloric acid (HCl) [5]. This test showed that hydrolyzed collagen guarantees a consistent and dose-dependent barrier effect against high concentration of HCl, which correlated with the molecular weight and amino acid composition of the protein. As a matter of fact, partially hydrolyzed collagen (molecular weight 5.000–10.000 Da) was about fivefold more potent than totally hydrolyzed collagen (molecular weight 1.000–3.000 Da), whereas the different aminoacidic composition of bovine and fish collagen reflects a greater barrier effect for the latter.

The trophic effect of collagen overlaps the mechanistic one. It is typically used in cell cultures. For example, an addition of collagen to the culture medium enhances exponentially the growth rate of the fibroblast subpopulation [6]. This property of collagen is typically used in the wound healing management, taking part in the proliferative and maturation phases, leading to the epithelization of the damage tissue. In human living, the aforementioned actions are interconnected. In fact, after the mechanistic action, collagen disintegrates, nourishing the surrounding tissues with the products of this disruption, peptides, and free amino acids [7, 8].

2. Metabolism of collagen in human body

The metabolism of collagen in the mammalian organism must take into account not only the molecular structure of collagen, but also its relation to other constituents of the tissue of which it is a part. Concerning the metabolic turnover of collagen, studies have shown that it is daily exposed on one side to a continuous loss, on the other side to an equally continuous newly synthesis. Nevertheless, when the loss overcomes the newly synthesis of collagen, it springs into a nosographic condition, comparable to avitaminosis, namely collagen carential disease [9]. Of the several conditions in which collagen structure or metabolism is disrupted, these changes lead to two pathological conditions: these are scurvy and lathyrism [10].

The loss of collagen is due both to the degradation implicit in the structural functions of the protein and to the products of its metabolism, which disperse outside the organism through the main route of elimination. The rate of the aforementioned loss has not been precisely determined, but its magnitude can be deduced from the daily protein requirement. It is in the order of 0.8 g/kg/day or about 55 g daily [11, 12]: in the organism collagen represents from 25 to 35% of the whole protein content [13], it derives a requirement of about 0.2–03 g/kg/day, corresponding to 14–18 g daily. This is the rate of the loss of collagen involved in the collagen carential disease.

Furthermore, pyridinoline (PYD) and deoxypyridinoline (DPD) are bone cross-linking compound of collagen fibers. PYD and DPD are formed during collagen maturation, thus their presence in both serum and urine is the result of collagen degradation, representing a useful diagnostic tool for the collagen carential disease.

Concerning the process of newly synthesis of collagen, it must be considered that collagen is a protein and, unlike vitamins and other essential nutrients, cannot be introduced into the organism as such. If it happened, collagen would trigger an immune, potentially auto-disruptive, reaction. Therefore, the focus shifts from the collagen itself to the raw materials required for its synthesis, which mainly consist of peptides and free amino acids.

Limited to nonessential amino acids, the raw material is partly synthesized ex novo inside the organism, whereas the remainder is recycled from preexisting proteins. Nevertheless, the main source is presumably represented by the products of food digestion. The last way is the most relevant, depending merely on food supply and supplementation.

Typically, a balanced diet should guarantee the adequate supply of amino acids necessary to synthesize collagen to maintain its homeostasis across the human body. However, there are critical issues that deserve attention. Firstly, collagen has a unique amino acid composition, which is made up of 20 amino acids. Of the nine amino acids designed as essential for human body, only methionine is slightly present and tryptophan is completely absent. Typical for collagen is the presence of essential amino acids, but also modified amino acids, namely 3-hydroxyproline, 4-hydroxyproline, and 5-hydroxyproline. Collagen also contains carbohydrate units, linked to hydroxylysine residues via the hydroxyl functional group of the amino acid. Gly and Pro in collagen structure are at 10–20-fold concentration found in other proteins. In order to ingest the same amount of glycine that is contained in 10 g of gelatin, one would have to consume about 2.8 L of milk or 160 g of meat. In the case of proline, the equivalent amounts are 0.4 L and 110 g, respectively [4]. For this reason, the amino acid composition of collagen has no significant correspondence in other proteins, neither animal nor vegetable. Therefore, the protein dietary intake can help, but it is not enough. Moreover, beyond certain limits, it takes negative effects, favoring the urinary elimination of calcium, the absorption of undigested proteins, and the accumulation of toxic portions [14–16].

In essence, the only protein that guarantees a correct amino acids supply for the endogenous synthesis of collagen is collagen itself, except that it is slightly digestible.

In this way, we have arrived to talk about hydrolyzed collagen (HC), also known as gelatin, which is progressively affirming in the treatment of the collagen carential disease. Gelatin is typically obtained from type I bovine skin collagen and from type I fish skin collagen. In brief, the skin of the animal is cleansed and treated with alkali and acid to prepare it to the extraction process. It was done by increasing the temperature of water till boiling. Then, collagen was in water solution ready to be purified using ultrafiltration and ionic exchange resins. After that, the solution is concentrated under vacuum, to reach the right concentration for the drying step. Apart from acids and alkalis, enzymes, or a combination of enzymes and chemicals, are also used for cleaving the cross-links. Special proteolytic enzymes are used as pepsin, neutrase, alkalase, bromelain, or papain. The selection of enzyme(s) and hydrolysis conditions essentially determine the sensory properties of the final product. Lastly, gelatin is spray-dried to a powder [5].

This "pre-digestion" promotes the gastro-enteric digestion and absorption in the form of peptides and free amino acids, tripling the bioavailability of collagen [17–19]. Orally administered gelatin is digested in the gut, crosses the intestinal barrier, becoming available for the metabolic process in the tissues. It has been proposed that HC peptides are only digested reaching the blood by passing through the enterocyte (transcytosis) at a level of approximately 10% [20].

3. Medical uses of hydrolyzed collagen via the oral and topical route

The term collagen derives from Greek κόλλα, meaning "glue," and suffix -γέν, –gen, denoting "producing." In fact, as early 3000 years ago, Egyptians used collagen solution as a biological glue to repair wooden articles. However, around 1800 A.D., collagen had its real development, being used as the main protein source in the diet of the French population who, due to the port blocks imposed by the British fleet, found themselves deprived of meat. The empiric uses of gelatin, for health protection, are widely documented since the Middle Age. Hildegard von Bingen was a German Benedictine abbess active as a writer, philosopher, composer, and medical writer during the High Middle Ages. In her book "Physica," dated around 1150 A.D., she recommended frequent and abundant meals of broth produced with veal fragments, very rich in collagen, to give well-being to joint pain.

The first therapeutic application of hydrolyzed collagen dates back to the second half of the last century, when in the United States it was mainly used to treat affections of the skin appendages, which typically concerned nail weakness, improving nail growth and strength. Hence, the idea to use HC in a method for treating disorders of the scalp, such as thinning or fall of hair. In 1976, Scala et al. did not observe an effect from HC treatment on the growth of hair, but it was due to the short duration of treatment, which was 4–8 weeks for the cat and dog. In the patent titled "Method for treatment of disorders of the piliferous system in mammals," the author reported that the administration of gelatin in the dosage of 100–500 mg/Kg increases the growth of hair in the rat, the dog, the rabbit, and the cat [21]. After due consideration to the different life span between these animal species and human, it was considered appropriate a period of three months' administration of 8–16 g of gelatin per day in order to obtain important results in the hair growth in human [22]. Thus, we arrive in 1998 when the use of hydrolyzed collagen was described for the preparation of food supplements, as a source of essential amino acids for the trophism of the scalp and the treatment of dystrophic disease in humans and animals [17].

Clinically, the signs and symptoms of the collagen carential disease present a dystrophic-degenerative character. The pathological conditions due to its deficiency involve, practically, the whole organism, based on the ancient criterion ex juvantibus, which dates back to the diagnosis of a disease through its treatment. As a matter of fact, this criterion has been used to diagnose avitaminosis and the other deficiency pathologies so far known. We can find the clearest expression of collagen carential disease in the osteoarticular, cutaneous, and mucous systems, nowadays the most documented systems.

Several scientific studies have demonstrated that a diet containing gelatin can improve the structure and health of the skin, bone, hair, and fingernails. Osteoarthritis is one of the main joint diseases, characterized by breakdown of joint cartilage and underlying bone. Its degeneration causes pain, lower mobility, and decrease of the quality of life. The main goal of prevention and treatment of osteoarthritis is related to decrease the degradation of joint cartilage, protecting it from further damage. The chondrocytes, the main cellular elements of cartilage, have to be supplied with structural elements necessary during the renewal phase. The administration of substances that are capable of supporting the cartilage with suitable nutrients promotes the cartilage to regenerate itself. Jiang et al. confirmed that hydrolyzed collagen improves joint health in patients with osteoarthritis. A prospective, randomized, double-blind, placebo-controlled study was performed in elderly woman with moderate knee osteoarthritis, and it showed that oral intake of gelatin for 6 months significantly reduces joint pain, improving mobility as assessed by two well-established scoring system (WOMAC and Lysholm score) [23].

Osteoporosis, like osteoarthritis, is a worldwide disease. It reduces drastically the bone density and the bone's structure becomes porous and weak, decreasing the capacity of bones to guarantee their structural function. Osteoporosis is easier to prevent than to treat. Typically, its prophylaxis and treatment are based on supplies of calcium. However, the primary structural element of bone is collagen, and the loss of minerals also means increased loss of collagen. This can be measured by analyzing the urine. By administering collagen hydrolysate, the building blocks required for renewing bone collagen are provided, and the body then uses them for this purpose [4]. To date, many clinical studies have evaluated its effects on bone metabolism. In most studies, hydrolyzed collagen is applied in association with other drugs, whereas in other studies, it is used as a single therapeutic element. In a first study, Adam et al. showed the effects of calcitonin, alone or in combination with a hydrolyzed collagen, on bone metabolism in postmenopausal women. The results underlined that a daily ingestion of 10 g of hydrolyzed collagen, in association with intramuscular injection of calcitonin (100 UI) twice a week for 24 weeks, enhanced and prolonged the effect of the drug as shown by a fall in urinary pyridinoline cross-link levels [20].

In a prospective, randomized, double-blind, placebo-controlled study, postmenopausal woman received 5 g/daily of collagen peptides for 12 months to evaluate its effects on bone mineral density (BMD) of the lower spine and the femoral neck. Daily intake of collagen reflected a positive shift in bone markers. As a matter of fact, the amino-terminal propeptide of type 1 procollagen (P1NP) significantly increased in the study group, indicating a stimulation of bone formation, whereas no changes in bone degradation markers could be determined. BMD increased significantly in the spine (3%) and in the femoral neck (6.7%), whereas no significant changes were determined in the placebo group [24].

Regarding the effects of hydrolyzed collagen on cutaneous diseases, 89 patients with stage II, III, or IV pressure ulcers were enrolled in a double-blinded, placebo controlled, randomized, multicenter trial. Hydrolyzed collagen intake was provided for 8 weeks at the dose of 15 g in a 45-mL unit dose. For the first time, results indicate that orally administration of hydrolyzed collagen can promote healing of pressure ulcers in addition with standard care [25]. Additionally, the oral administration of gelatin increased skin hydration after 8 weeks of supplementation; whereas ex vivo experiments demonstrated that collagen peptides induce collagen as well as glycosaminoglycan production [26]. This is due to its amino acid composition that activates the synthesis of collagen and glycosaminoglycan in the human body. Furthermore, hydrolyzed collagen helps to improve the strength and hardness of nails and hair. For instance, in one study, based on 14 g/daily diet of gelatin treatment for three months, the mean hair diameter increased by an average of 10%. Increases in the size of the hair stalk and the hair density were also reported as noted in a three-month application study, fingernails became firmer and less brittle [4]. Hexsel et al. investigated the daily ingestion of hydrolyzed collagen for 24 weeks increasing nail growth and improving brittle nails with a notable decrease in the frequency of broken nails [27], whereas Chen et al. found the essential relationships between collagen and hair follicle regeneration. It confirmed that collagen could be a therapeutic target for hair loss as well as skin-related diseases [28].

Recently, the medical use of collagen has also been extended to gastric diseases [29, 30]. two pathogenetic factors play an important role in dyspepsia: an excessive secretion of hydrochloric acid by parietal cells and a reduction of the mucus that covers and protects the internal surface of the stomach. Ulcerative forms from non-steroidal anti-inflammatory drugs (NSAIDs) are a typical example of the second factor, resulting in part from the reduction of prostaglandin activity, in part from a contact action, which occurs locally on the gastrointestinal wall. Antacids and antisecretors, particularly the proton pump inhibitors (PPIs), have found to be important in the treatment of dyspepsia, but they are displaying some unwanted toxicity that limits their use. It is due to a drastic reduction of gastric acidity, which decreases digestibility and absorption of essential nutrients, representing a risk factor for cognitive decline, such as suggested in recent observational studies and systemic reviews of the literature. Moreover, the excessive reduction of stomach pH increases the vulnerability to infection. As such, there is an emerging interest in developing medications to treat dyspepsia not by reducing gastric acidity, but by increasing mucosal protection toward hydrochloric acid. This approach thus preserves the positive effects of sterilization, digestion, and absorption of food [5]. Hydrolyzed collagen is a main candidate, showing both a mechanistic action, which protects as a biological veil the gastric mucosa against hydrochloric acid injury, then a trophic one, nourishing and regenerating the suffering mucosa.

International Patent US 10,973,850 discloses a novel composition comprising tricalcium phosphate and gelatin for use in a method for the treatment of dyspepsia and related disorders [29].

Furthermore, United States Food and Drug Administration recently approved the use of Hemospray, a collagen powder administered through endoscopy, for the management of GI bleeding [30].

Thus, we arrive to talk about another property of collagen, that is, its involvement in platelet adhesion and activation, triggering phase of the coagulation. As a matter of fact, when the endothelium is damaged, collagen is exposed to circulating platelets, which bind directly to collagen through collagen-specific glycoprotein Ia/IIa surface receptors. This bound is strengthened by von Willebrand factor (vWF), which is released from platelets and from the endothelium. These interactions lead to the platelet activation, which changes shape from discoidal to spherical, favoring the aggregation process to the site of injury. Collagen also accelerates reparative processes and initiates wound healing through activation of inflammatory cells and tissue vascularization. Collagen has also been shown to stimulate angiogenic growth factors and epithelial cell migration and proliferation, leading to re-epithelialization [31].

In addition to the oral supplementation, hydrolyzed collagen also manifests its biological effects by topical route. Fore et al. concluded that the use of a topical hydrolyzed collagen is an acceptable adjunct therapy for the treatment of Pyoderma gangrenosum (PG) lesions. A topical mixture of hydrolyzed collagen powder with equal volumes of 4 mg/ml dexamethasone phosphate liquid and 40 mg/ml gentamycin liquid compounded to a paste consistency was applied to the wound, with additional application of a compression dressing once a week. The lesions are healed in 4 months. Hydrolyzed collagen helps granulation and epithelization acting as an absorbable reservoir for anti-inflammatory and antimicrobial agents. The association of hydrolyzed collagen and antibiotic agents provides an effective topical treatment for this hard wound [32].

In recent years, collagen has found widespread para-pharmaceutical uses, typically in the form of food supplements, cosmetics, and medical devices, with defined physiological effects and without adverse reaction. Of particular interest is the use of HC for skin through topical application, in consideration of the physiological role recognized to this apparatus. The skin performs functions of protection, self-repair, thermoregulation, control, secretion, absorption, and sensory activity. According to a recent discovery, moreover, it acts as a solar panel. Unlike photovoltaics, it does not turn light into simple electricity, which requires complex processes to translate into a consumer product. The skin is capable of transforming solar power directly into hormones, vitamins, neurotransmitters, and other products crucial to the functioning of the skin per se, but also for the whole body including different organs. Indeed, these new observations provide explanation of more complex phenomena, such as the correlation between mood and sun exposure [33].

The Ehlers-Danlos syndrome (EDS) describes another group of genetic collagen disorders, affecting the collagen processing and structure. It is a rare disorder comprising a group of related inherited disorders of connective tissue, resulting from underlying abnormalities in the synthesis and metabolism of collagen, which is characterized by joint hypermobility and susceptibility to arthritis, skin, and vascular problems. EDS occurs due to variations of more than 19 genes that are present at birth. The specific gene affected determines the type of EDS. Actually, no cure is known, and the treatment is only a palliative one. Physical therapy and bracing may help strengthen muscles and support joint [34].

The novel aspect proposed in this work is that its pathogenesis once thought to result from defective genes alone could be influenced, in some cases, by food deficiencies, which in the case of Ehlers-Danlos syndrome concern the amino acids suitable for the endogenous synthesis of collagen. In essence, nutrient deficiencies could unmask and highlight the underlying genetic malformations; in the same way food supplement could be a valid aid not only for the containment and prevention of these diseases but also as a treatment. Likewise, it is known that spina bifida is caused by a combination of genetic and nutritional factors. Whereas it is produced by an acid folic deficiency during pregnancy, a dietary supplementation of folic acid has been shown to reduce the incidence of spina bifida.

Hence, the idea of an "extended collagen carential disease," applicable to the absence of essential nutritional factors in the Ehlers-Danlos syndrome, plays an important role in the pathogenesis and treatment of genetic diseases.

4. Conclusion

In conclusion, collagen is a family of proteins present in the whole organism, linking its parts and carrying out precise physiological roles. The tropocollagen, a protein of about 300 kDa genetically predetermined, is its progenitor and carrier. The various types of collagens, which characterize its presence and tangible functions in the body, take shape after an essentially posttranscriptional process. Around the backbone of tropocollagen, XXVIII different types of collagens take shape, with essentially posttranslational modalities. After its biosynthesis by fibroblasts and their subpopulations, the tropocollagen is glycosylated in the Golgi apparatus. Then it goes outside the cell. Through cross-links and the assumption of other molecules by Van der Waals forces, it takes the definitive conformations that distinguish its functions in the single organs and tissues. The tropocollagen represents, therefore, the common matrix and the unifying element of the variegated collagen typology.

Collagen has two distinct but interconnected properties: first, a mechanistic effect of support and protection; second, a trophic effect that nourishes the tissues, favoring the production of new collagen. Collagen is also subject to an important turnover, due both to its catabolism and to the end products of its biological cycle poured out in the form of hairs, desquamations, and secretions. This cycle, if not adequately integrated with components from the outside, results in a deficit of collagen leading to the collagen carential disease.

Our organism reproduces collagen at the expense of the amino acids obtained from food or newly synthesized. A high-protein diet can help in the treatment of collagen carential disease, but is not enough, mainly for the particular amino acid composition of collagen, which does not match in other proteins. The only protein capable of ensuring a correct amino acids supply would be native collagen, except that it is not digestible. The solution is offered by hydrolyzed collagen, which is more digestible and ingestible than the native one.

Twenty years ago, a famous physiologist stated that the understanding of the physiology of collagen was rudimentary [1]. In the meantime, a huge amount of knowledge has accumulated, opening the way to the treatment of the "collagen carential disease," with involves the whole organism. This chapter draws attention on the Ehlers-Danlos syndrome, suggesting a carential role aside the genetic one.

Author details

Bruno Silvestrini[1]*, Chuen Yan Cheng[2] and Matteo Innocenti[1]

1 Noopolis Foundation, Rome, Italy

2 Population Council, Center for Biomedical Research, New York, USA

*Address all correspondence to: brunosilvestrini25@gmail.com

References

[1] Rennie M. Teasing out the truth about collagen. The Journal of Physiology. 1999;**521**(Pt 1 (Pt 1)):1. DOI: 10.1111/j.1469-773.1999.00001.x

[2] Minor RR. Collagen metabolism: A comparison of diseases of collagen and diseases affecting collagen. The American Journal of Pathology. 1980; **98**(1):225-280

[3] Peterkofsky B. Ascorbate requirement for hydroxylation and secretion of procollagen: Relationship to inhibition of collagen synthesis in scurvy. The American Journal of Clinical Nutrition. 1991;**54**(Suppl. 6):1135S-1140S. DOI: 10.1093/ajcn/54.6.1135s

[4] Schrieber R, Gareis H. Gelatine Handbook-Theory and Industrial Practice. Weinheim: WILEY-VCH Verlag GmbH & Co. KGaA; 2007

[5] Silvestrini B, Silvestri R, Cheng CY, Ceracchi M, Innocenti M. A method to measure the barrier effect of drug and its application in the study of hydrolyzed collagen. Agro Food Industry Hi Tech. 2021;**32**(3):12-16

[6] Themistocleous GS, Katopodis H, Sourla A, Lembessis P, Doillon CJ, Soucacos PN, et al. Three-dimensional type I collagen cell culture systems for the study of bone pathophysiology. In Vivo. 2004;**18**(6):687-696

[7] Postlethwaite AE, Seyer JM, Kang AH. Chemotactic attraction of human fibroblasts to type I, II, and III collagens and collagen-derived peptides. Proceedings of the National Academy of Sciences of the United States of America. 1978;**75**(2):871-875

[8] Shigemura Y, Iwai K, Morimatsu F, Iwamoto T, Mori T, Oda C, et al. Effect of prolyl-hydroxyproline (Pro-Hyp), a food-derived collagen peptide in human blood, on growth of fibroblasts from mouse skin. Journal of Agricultural and Food Chemistry. 2009;**57**(2):444

[9] Silvestrini B, Innocenti M, Perrotta AM, Cheng CY. Physiopathology and treatment of collagen carential disease. Minerva Medica. 2019;**112**(3):403-404. DOI: 10.23736/S0026-4806.19.06036-1

[10] William Van B. Robertson: Metabolism of collagen in mammalian tissues. Biophysical Journal. 1964;**4**(1 Pt 2):93-106. DOI: 10.1016/s0006-3495(64)86930-7

[11] National Research Council (US) Subcommittee on the Tenth Edition of the Recommended Dietary Allowances. Recommended Dietary Allowances: 10th Edition. Washington (DC): National Academies Press (US); 1989. PMID: 25144070

[12] Waterlow JC. Metabolic adaptation to low intakes of energy and protein. Annual Review of Nutrition. 1986;**6**:495-526. DOI: 10.1146/annurev.nu.06070186.002431

[13] Di Lullo GA, Sweeney SM, Korkko J, Ala-Kokko L, San Antonio JD. Mapping the ligand-binding sites and disease-associated mutations on the most abundant protein in the human, type I collagen. The Journal of Biological Chemistry. 2002;**277**(6):4223-4231. DOI: 10.1074/jbc.M110709200

[14] Ameye LG, Chee WSS. Osteoarthritis and nutrition. From nutraceuticals to functional foods: A systematic review

of the scientific evidence. Arthritis Research & Therapy. 2006;**8**(4):R127. DOI: 10.1186/ar2016

[15] Berg RA, Kerr JS. Nutritional aspects of collagen metabolism. Annual Review of Nutrition. 1992;**12**:369-390. DOI: 10.1146/annurev.nu.12.070192.002101

[16] Cooper C, Atkinson EJ, Hensrud DD, Wahner HW, O'Fallon WM, Riggs BL, et al. Dietary protein intake and bone mass in women. Calcified Tissue International. 1996;**58**(5):320-325. DOI: 10.1007/BF02509379

[17] Silvestrini B, Gunter K: Integratori alimentari e dietetici contenenti gelatina idrolizzata e loro uso in campo medico sanitario. 1998; IT1299131 (B1)

[18] Ichikawa S, Morifuji M, Ohara H, Matsumoto H, Takeuchi Y, Sato K. Hydroxyproline-containing dipeptides and tripeptides quantified at high concentration in human blood after oral administration of gelatin hydrolysate. International Journal of Food Science and Nutrition. 2010;**61**(1):1-9. DOI: 10.3109/096374809 03257711

[19] Taga Y, Kusubata M, Ogawa-Goto K, Hattori S. Identification of collagen-derived hydroxyproline (Hyo)-containing cyclic dipeptides with high oral bioavailability: efficient formation of cyclo (X-Hyp) from X-Hyp-Gly-Type tripeptides by heating. Journal of Agricultural and Food Chemistry. 2020;**14**:43. DOI: 10.1021/acs.jafc.7b03714

[20] Daneault A, Prawitt J, Soulé VF, Coxam V, Wittran Y. Biological effect of hydrolyzed collagen on bone metabolism. Critical Reviews in Food Science and Nutrition. 2017;**57**(9):1922-1937. DOI: 10.1080/10408398.2015.1038377

[21] Silvestrini B. Metodo per il trattamento di disturbi del sistema pilifero in mammiferi. 1986; Patent IT 1135585

[22] Silvestrini B. Method for increasing hair growth. 1988; Patent n° 4,749,684

[23] Jiang J-X, Yu S, Huang Q-R, Zhang X-L, Zhang C-Q, Zhou J-L, et al. Collagen peptides improve knee osteoarthritis in elderly women: A 6-month randomized, double-blind, placebo-controlled study. Agro Food Industry Hi Tech. 2014;**25**(2):19-23

[24] König D, Oesser S, Scharla S, Zdzieblik D, Gollhofer A. Specific collagen peptides improve bone mineral density and bone markers in postmenopausal women—A randomized controlled study. Nutrients. 2018;**10**(1):97. DOI: 10.3390/nu10010097

[25] Kwon Lee S, Posthauer ME, Dorner B, Redovian V, Maloney MJ. Pressure ulcer healing with a concentrated, fortified, collagen protein hydrolysate supplement: A randomized controlled trial. Advances in Skin & Wound Care: The Journal for Prevention and Healing. 2006;**19**(2):92-96

[26] Asserin J, Lati E, Shioya T, Prawitt J. The effect of oral collagen peptide supplementation on skin moisture and dermal collagen network: Evidence from an ex vivo model and randomized, placebo-controlled clinical trials. Journal of Cosmetic Dermatology. 2015;**14**:291-301. DOI: 10.1111/jocd.12174

[27] Hexsel D, Zague V, Shunck M, Siega C, Comozzato FO, Oesser S. Oral supplementation with specific bioactive collagen peptides improves nail growth and reduces symptoms of brittle nails. Journal of Cosmetic Dermatology. 2017;**16**(4):520-526. DOI: 10.1111/jocd.12393

[28] Chen P, Cescon M, Bonaldo P. Lack of collagen VI promotes wound-induced hair growth. The Journal of Investigative Dermatology. 2015;**135**(10):2358-2367. DOI: 10.1038/jid.2015.187

[29] Silvestrini B. Composition comprising tricalcium phosphate and gelatin for use in a method for the treatment of dyspepsia and related disorders. US 10,973,850 B2. 2021

[30] Bansal RK, Gupta MK, Gupta VK, Kaur G, Seth AK. Endoscopic treatment of upper gastrointestinal bleeding using Haemoseal spray: A retrospective, observational study from a tertiary center in north India. Journal of Digestive Endoscopy. 2020;**11**:279-282. DOI: 10.1055/s-0040-1722387

[31] Key N, Makris M, O'Shaughnessy D, Lillicrap D. Practical Hemostasis and Thrombosis. 2nd ed. USA: Wiley-Blackwell; 2008. p. 2

[32] Fore J, Zinszer KM, Patel UK, Vetti LTP. A novel topical therapy for Pyoderma Gangrenosum using compounded hydrolyzed type I bovine collagen. Case report 26th Annual Clinical Symposium on Advances in Skin & Wound Care, National Harbor | September 9-12, 2011

[33] Silvestrini B. La cosmesi moderna: da arte della bellezza a scienza medica. HPC Today. 2021;**16**(1):14-17

[34] Mantle D, Wilkins RM, Preedy V. A novel therapeutic strategy for Ehlers–Danlos syndrome based on nutritional supplements. Medical Hypotheses. 2005;**64**(2):279-283. DOI: 10.1016/j.mehy.2004.07.023

Chapter 2

Supercritical Carbon Dioxide Facilitated Collagen Scaffold Production for Tissue Engineering

Periasamy Srinivasan and Dar-Jen Hsieh

Abstract

The rise of tissue engineering and regenerative medicine (TERM) is a developing field that focuses on the advancement of alternative therapies for tissue and organ restoration. Collagen scaffold biomaterials play a vital role as a scaffold to promote cell growth and differentiation to promote the repair and regenerate the tissue lesion. The goal of this chapter will be to evaluate the role of supercritical carbon dioxide extraction technology in the production of collagen scaffold biomaterials from various tissues and organs and relate it to the traditional decellularization techniques in the production of collagen biomaterials for TERM. Therefore, we will study the collagen scaffold biomaterials produced using supercritical carbon dioxide extraction technology and their characteristics, such as chemical-physical properties, toxicity, biocompatibility, *in vitro* and *in vivo* bioactivity that could affect the interaction with cells and living system, relative to traditional decellularization technique-mediated collagen scaffolds. Furthermore, the chapter will focus on supercritical carbon dioxide extraction technology for the production of collagen scaffolds biomaterial appropriate for TERM.

Keywords: supercritical carbon dioxide extraction technology, tissue engineering, regenerative medicine, biomaterial, collagen scaffold, biocompatibility

1. Introduction

Tissue engineering advanced from the field of biomaterials development and denotes the practice of combining cells, tissue scaffolds, and bioactive signal molecules. These tissue scaffolds are produced by various decellularization processes, such as chemical and physical methods. Tissue scaffolds, cells, and biologically active signal molecules are the three key elements for tissue and organ reparation. Tissue engineering is defined as "*an interdisciplinary field of research that applies the principles of engineering and the life science toward the development of biological substitutes that restore, maintain or improve tissue function*" [1]. Regenerative medicine is a wide field that comprises tissue engineering but also integrates research on self-healing in which the body uses its systems, sometimes with help of foreign biological material to reconstruct and rebuild tissues and organs. The terms tissue engineering and "regenerative medicine" have become largely interchangeable, as the field hopes to focus on cures as an alternative for the treatment of complex, mainly chronic diseases (e.g. Diabetic wound healing, burn wounds).

2. Tissue engineering and regenerative medicine

Tissue engineering and regenerative medicine (TERM) have been projected and established for almost 30 years. Though many fruitful challenges in tissue regeneration have been attained, TERM is still in its infancy stage and most of the vital questions remain to be answered, including the selection of cell sources, development of tissue-specific materials, and construction of complex organs. The most important is the *in vivo* mechanism of the formation of new tissue and organ employing the tissue-engineered biomaterials, and the process to resemble and transform to native tissue and organ. The subsequent transformation and final destination of the biomaterials remain to be the serious apprehensions in this dynamically emerging field. Addressing these queries is significant to the effectiveness, stability, and security of the clinical application of tissue-engineered biomaterials [2].

Tissue and organ repair remain a clinical issue and challenge. Entirely restoring or regenerating damaged tissues and organs and reestablishing their functions have been a vision of medical society. The emergence of tissue engineering and regenerative medicine (TERM) makes it possible. TERM is a developing field that focuses on the advancement of alternative therapies for tissue and organ restoration [2, 3]. TERM is an extremely multidisciplinary arena, in which bioengineering and medicine unite. It is constructed on integrative approaches using scaffolds, cells, growth factors, nanomedicine, and other techniques to pass on the restrictions that presently exist in the hospitals. Certainly, TERM overall aim is to encourage the formation of new functional tissues, rather than just implanting tissue and bone parts [2]. TERM is a multifaceted science and associates basic sciences such as materials science, biomechanics, cell biology, and medical sciences to comprehend functional tissue and organ restoration and reconstruction. The world's population is aging and the trend is escalating. There is a severe global shortage of tissues and organs for transplantation. TERM has the potential to meet the requirements of the forthcoming needs of patients [2, 4]. TERM aims to create a three-dimensional (3D) cell-biomaterial composite, that possesses a comparable function as living tissue and organ and is employed to restore or regenerate damaged tissue and organ. The basic condition for the 3D composite is to support cell growth, nutrition and waste transport and gas exchange. TERM typically employs the following strategies, cell-biomaterial composite, in which cell-seeded biomaterials are implanted into the body to restore and regenerate tissues and organs; stem cell transplantation; and biomaterial implanted into the body and undertake the process of tissue integration [3]. Scaffolds are vital for tissue engineering approaches for several reasons; as a three-dimensional structure, they offer volume fill, mechanical integrity and a surface that can afford chemical and architectural guidance for regenerating tissues [5]. The three vital elements in TERM are cells, scaffolds and signals (**Figure 1**). Several decellularization techniques had been used for the production of collagen scaffolds for TERM application, including the supercritical carbon dioxide ($SCCO_2$) extraction technology to be discussed here in this article.

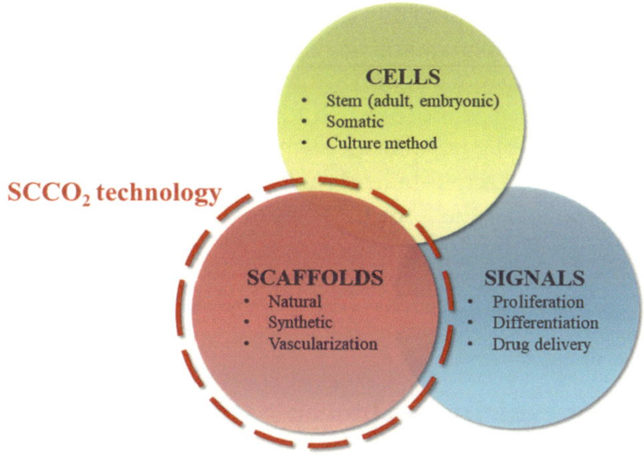

Figure 1.
The triad of TERM.

3. Collagen scaffolds-biomaterial for TERM

Collagen-based biomaterial application in the field of TERM has been significantly increasing over the past decades. Collagen owns the main advantages as it is biodegradable, biocompatible, easily available and highly versatile. However, collagen is a protein, therefore it is problematic to sterilize without altering its native structure. Collagen-based biomaterials developed for TERM were intended to provide a functional biomaterial for use in TERM from the laboratory bench to the patient bedside [6]. Collagen is present in all connective tissue and makes it one of the most studied biomolecules of the extracellular matrix (ECM). It is the major component of skin and bone and constitutes approximately 25–35% of mammalian total dry weight [7]. Until

Type	Molecular formula	Form	Distribution
I	$[\alpha1(I)]_2\alpha2(I)$	Fibril	Bone, skin, tendons, ligaments, cornea
II	$[\alpha1(II)]_3$	Fibril	Cartilage, intervertebral disc, notochord, vitreous humor in the eye
III	$[\alpha1(III)]_3$	Fibril	Skin, blood vessels
V	$[\alpha1(V)]_2\alpha2(V)$ and $\alpha1(V)\alpha2(V)\alpha3(V)$	Fibril (assemble with type I)	*idem* as type I
XI	$\alpha1(XI)\alpha2(XI)\alpha3(XI)$	Fibril (assemble with type II)	*idem* as type II
IX	$\alpha1(IX)\alpha2(IX)\alpha3(IX)$	Lateral association with type II fibril	Cartilage
XII	$[\alpha1(XII)]_3$	Lateral association with type I fibril	Tendons, ligaments
IV	$[\alpha1(IV)]_2\alpha2(IV)$	Sheet-like network	Basal lamina
VII	$[\alpha1(VII)]_3$	Anchoring fibrils	Beneath stratified squamous epithelia

Table 1.
Collagen types, forms and distribution [6].

now, 29 diverse collagen genotypes have been characterized and all depict a typical triple helix structure. Fiber form of collagens are types I, II, III, V and XI. Collagen molecules are made up of three α chains that assemble due to their molecular structure. Each α chain is made up of more than a 1000 amino acids based on the repeated sequence -Gly-X-Y-. The vital part is the presence of glycine at every third amino acid position to permit for a tight triple-helical packaging of the three α polypeptide chains. In the tropocollagen molecule the X and Y positions are mostly filled by proline and 4-hydroxyproline [6, 7]. Though numerous types of collagens (**Table 1**) have been defined, only a few types are used to yield collagen-based biomaterials. Currently, type I collagen is the gold standard in the field of TERM.

4. Collagen immunogenicity and biocompatibility

Medical application of collagen biomaterial needs to make a clear difference between immunogenicity and antigenicity. Immunogenicity is triggering an immune response; however, antigenicity denotes the interaction between the antibodies and the antigenic epitopes. Collagen mediated immune response primarily targets epitopes in the telopeptide region at each end of the tropocollagen molecule. The polymerized collagen fibrils conformity of the helical part and the amino acid sequence on the surface can influence the immunologic profile of the collagen molecule [7]. Type I collagen is an appropriate biomaterial for implantation meanwhile only an insignificant number of people have humoral immunity against type I collagen. In addition, a simple serologic test can validate an allergic reaction in response to type I collagen-based biomaterial. It is most crucial to discuss that collagen immunogenicity which is relevant to collagen molecules that are made up of an acellular ECM and the utmost adverse immune responses that have been come across with an acellular scaffold are not necessarily initiated from the collagen molecule itself. Incomplete decellularization with the presence of remaining oligosaccharide α-Gal and DNA is the common reason for acute immune responses and subsequent acellular ECM rejection [7, 8].

5. Traditional decellularization of tissues and organs for collagen biomaterial

The traditional decellularization techniques involve long duration and increased cost as well as long-term washing of the tissue material from the residual and traces of the chemicals used. Despite the numerous decellularization process that exists, it is necessary to go through a lot of parameters for multiple reasons in the decellularization process (**Table 2**). The decellularization process aims to remove the cellular material of the donor, antigens, and potential pathogens. In addition, the most critical issue is to offer the conservation of the structural organization of an ECM with the set of functions inherent in it. Therefore, the optimization of these decellularization methods and the pursuit of improved methods are still ongoing [9]. At present, numerous procedures for decellularization of tissues were employed that include the treatment by detergents such as sodium dodecyl sulfate (SDS), sodium deoxycholate, Triton X-100, etc., and treatment by enzymes such as trypsin, deoxyribonuclease (DNase), and ribonuclease (RNase). Other methods include alkali treatment, as well as cyclic freezing-thawing and high-pressure action up to 1 GPa, which have been tried (**Table 3**) [9, 23].

Decellularization techniques	Advantages	Disadvantages
Supercritical carbon dioxide extraction technology	Supercritical phase pressure disrupts ECM. Uses inert gas (CO_2) for cell removal and do not alter ECM's mechanical properties	No known disadvantages. Not yet widely employed for decellularization
Acids and bases (sulfuric acid, ammonium hydroxide, acetic acid, peracetic acid)	Disinfects material by entering inside microorganisms and oxidizing enzymes	Dissociate important molecules in ECM including GAGs, from collagen scaffold
Enzymes (trypsin)	Better preservation of GAG content	Disruptive to elastin and collagen and elicits immune response
Non-ionic detergents (Triton X-100)	Preserves protein-protein interactions intact and retains sulphated GAG content	Disrupts ECM ultrastructure and owers laminins/fibronectin content
Ionic detergents (sodium dodecyl sulphate (SDS))	Effectively removes cells from the tissue	Disrupts protein-protein interactions and causes a decrease in GAG content and collagen integrity
Zwitterionic detergents (CHAPS and SB-10/SB-16)	Preserves native ECM	A high degree of protein denaturation
Solvents (alcohols and acetone)	No advantages	Crosslinks and precipitates proteins, including collagen
Sonication	Effective cell removal	Parameters are not well standardized
High-pressure gradient system	Effective cell removal	Ineffective for densely organized ECM tissues

Table 2.
Decellularization techniques used for tissues, organs and their advantages and disadvantages.

Area of application	Title	Authors	Significance
Bone regeneration	Development of a decellularized porcine bone graft by supercritical carbon dioxide extraction technology for bone regeneration.	Chen et al. [10]	Production and evaluation of biocompatibility of bone graft
Skin regeneration	Regenerative porcine dermal collagen matrix developed by supercritical carbon dioxide extraction technology: Role in accelerated wound healing.	Wang et al. [11]	Wound healing, skin graft and regeneration
Skincare industry and medical applications	Protocols for accelerated production and purification of collagen scaffold and atelocollagen from animal tissues.	Hsieh & Srinivasan [12]	Accelerated production and purification of atelocollagen
Experimental and clinical tissue regeneration	Protocols for the preparation and characterization of decellularized tissue and organ scaffolds for tissue engineering.	Hsieh et al. [13]	Preparation and characterization of decellularized tissue and organ scaffolds

Area of application	Title	Authors	Significance
Wound healing	Supercritical carbon dioxide-decellularized porcine acellular dermal matrix combined with autologous adipose-derived stem cells: Its role in accelerated diabetic wound healing.	Chou et al. [14]	Accelerated diabetic wound healing
Extraction socket bone regeneration	Evaluating the bone-regenerative role of the decellularized porcine bone xenograft in a canine extraction socket model.	Chen et al. [15]	Guided bone regeneration, extraction socket bone regeneration
Corneal replacement	Preparation of acellular scaffold for corneal tissue engineering by supercritical carbon dioxide extraction technology.	Huang et al. [16]	Production and evaluation of biocompatibility of acellular corneal scaffold
Bone regeneration	Reconstruction of the orbital floor using supercritical CO_2 decellularized porcine bone graft.	Huang et al. [17]	Orbital floor reconstruction
Corneal transplantation	Acellular porcine cornea produced by supercritical carbon dioxide extraction: A potential substitute for human corneal regeneration.	Liang et al. [18]	Biocompatibility of acellular corneal scaffold in rabbit lamellar corneal transplantation. Potential substitute for human-donated cornea for corneal transplantation
Bone regeneration	Supercritical carbon dioxide decellularized bone matrix seeded with adipose-derived mesenchymal stem cells accelerated bone regeneration.	Liu et al. [19]	Accelerated bone regeneration
Rhinoplasty	A novel 3D histotypic cartilage construct engineered by supercritical carbon dioxide decellularized porcine nasal cartilage graft and chondrocytes exhibited chondrogenic capability *in vitro*.	Lee et al. [20]	Engineered 3D histotypic cartilage construct for nasal septum reconstruction
Osteoarthritis	Supercritical carbon dioxide decellularized porcine cartilage graft with PRP attenuated OA progression and regenerated articular cartilage in ACLT-induced OA rats.	Wu et al. [21]	Repair and regeneration articular cartilage in osteoarthritis
Osteoarthritis	3D composite engineered using supercritical CO_2 decellularized porcine cartilage scaffold, chondrocytes, and PRP: Role in articular cartilage regeneration.	Chen et al. [22]	3D composite engineered decellularized porcine cartilage scaffold in articular cartilage regeneration

Table 3.
Porcine tissues and organs had been decellularized by the $SCCO_2$ process applied in different medical applications.

5.1 Tissues and organs

Currently, the most frequently employed decellularization technique for tissue and organ to manufacture scaffolds employing detergents are sodium dodecyl sulfate, Triton X-100, and CHAPS, branded as ionic, non-ionic, and zwitterionic detergents, respectively. Detergents were found to be effective in the decellularization of the tissues and organs, including the removal of lipids [24, 25]. Enzymes such as nucleases are also employed in limited decellularization protocols to eliminate the DNA from the tissues and organs [25, 26]. However, detergent-employed decellularization often disrupts the ECM by changing tertiary and quaternary structures of the proteins. SDS is known to proficiently eliminate glycosaminoglycans, thereby destructing the collagen structure [27]. Detergent decellularization is known to reduce the number of valuable growth factors that are vital for the recellularization of tissues. Moreover, residual surfactants and chemicals often cause cytotoxicity [28] inducing adverse effects in the recellularization of tissue and organ scaffolds (**Table 3**) [13, 26, 27].

5.2 Adipose tissue

Common traditional decellularization methods for adipose tissue include numerous freezing-thawing cycles, extraction of lipids with isopropanol, and enzymatic treatment. Developing a protocol for the preparation of ECM from adipose tissue in an accessible and eco-friendly manner will promote the upgrading of the methods of tissue engineering with the use of autologous material [9, 27, 29–31].

5.3 Pericardium

The existing techniques for pericardium decellularization include the treatment by non-ionic detergents such as Triton X-100, 3-3-chloroamidopropyl-dimethyl-ammonio-1-propanesulfonate (CHAPS), ionic detergents (SDS), sodium deoxycholate, alkalis, and enzymes such as trypsin with EDTA. However, the adverse effects are commonly occurred by the above-mentioned procedures on the ECM structure and composition. The detergents such as SDS and Triton X-100 were found to denature the collagen of the ECM which was elucidated by staining fluorescently labeled collagen hybridizing peptide. CHAPS and sodium deoxycholate altered the structural organization of collagen established by the recording of the second harmonic signal and transmission electron microscopy. Decellularization of bovine pericardium tissue using Triton X-100 reduces the concentration of glycosaminoglycans by ~62–66%, and in an alkaline solution, by ~88.6%, at the initial concentration of ~0.6 mg/g [9, 27, 29–31].

5.4 Bone

The current standard method employed for bone decellularization is by high-temperature sintering at 300–1300°C. Moreover, this procedure completely removes any possible zoonotic infectious agents, in addition to the immunogenic components that existed in the animal bone tissues [32]. However, the high-temperature sintering damages the intrinsic collagen and alters the porous ECM structures of the animal bones. Bone decellularization can also be carried out by various chemical agents and techniques. The chemical process includes processing the bone with acidic and alkaline solutions and organic agents, as well as detergents and enzymes, that unavoidably alter the ECM structure. Delipidation is the key factor in decellularization processing because indisputably, the residual lipids in the bone act as a barrier to cell removal, in addition to altering its biocompatibility and osseointegration [33]. Moreover, it encourages adverse reactions which can give rise to bone resorption and encapsulate fibrosis [10, 34].

5.5 Cartilage

Decellularization of cartilage is challenging, due to its dense structure with lacunae. Generally, decellularization of cartilage is performed by the perfusion of detergents into the lacunae to break down the chondrocytes. In continuation, the detergents were washed out of the residual cellular fragments and nucleic acids. In another case, decellularization of cartilage was performed by treating with 0.05% Trypsin/EDTA for 1 day followed by 3% SDS for 2 days and 3% Triton X-100 for another 2 days [35]. Decellularization of the cartilage process includes a mixture of physical, chemical, and enzymatic steps [35]. Decellularization of cartilage by SDS and Triton X-10 resulted in only a 77% decrease in DNA content (262 ± 42 ng/mg) relative to the untreated cartilage. But, the key norms for medical devices, the decellularized tissue residual DNA content should be less than 50 ng/mg in decellularized materials. However, the dense nature of the cartilages reticular network of fibrous ECM is a substantial barrier for the detergents to penetrate. It is the key limitation of SDS and Triton X-100 in cartilage decellularization [35, 36]. Cartilage complete decellularization by SDS (2%) treatment for 4 or 8 h; however, 60% of the DNA remained in the decellularized cartilage [20, 37]. Decellularization of cartilage by using 1% SDS for 24 h and 2% Triton X-100 for 48 h preserved most of the ECM components with a complete chondrocyte's removal. The complete decellularization of chondrocytes and the movement of seeded cells into the scaffolds during recellularization is challenging. The decellularization process in the SDS process caused the denaturation of proteins in ECM structures, which may also destroy the protein function [20, 38]. Cartilage decellularization methods such as chemical and enzymatic methods lead to disadvantages including traces of impurities and loss of ECM scaffold structure caused by the degradation of native collagen ECM structure leading to difficulty in the recellularization of the cartilage scaffold. Porcine articular cartilage decellularized by a succession of freeze-thaw cycles and 0.1–0.5% (w/v) sodium dodecyl sulfate detergent cycles with chondroitinase ABC and hyaluronidase were employed to breakdown glycosaminoglycans, resulting in the removal of 80–90% of the DNA [22, 39].

6. Supercritical carbon dioxide extraction technology, an innovative and efficient approach for collagen biomaterial production

The conditions necessary for the decellularization processing of biomaterials frequently reject the use of traditional approaches involving destructive action on the biomaterial such as high-temperature treatment, acid, and alkali, etc. A result of the search for an alternative process leads to novel processing technologies and approaches concentrating on the direction of green technology in the first place. Supercritical carbon dioxide extraction technology comes in the first place in green technology. Supercritical carbon dioxide extraction technology owns exceptional advantages that can be employed in the production of biomaterials efficiently and cost-effectively. The most vital and important advantage of $SCCO_2$ is the option of conducting processes at low temperatures, which offers the opportunity to work with a variety of biomaterials and thermally sensitive components such as collagen [40]. In the $SCCO_2$ process, the low surface tension encourages the penetration of CO_2 into solid and colloidal structures, which makes it competently decellularize and sterilize biomaterial and medical devices with the preservation of the structure and physicochemical properties (**Table 4**) [41].

In the supercritical process, the carbon dioxide gas above a critical temperature, Tc = 31.1°C, and pressure, Pc = 73.8 bar is said to be supercritical (**Figure 2**). In this state, carbon dioxide is neither a gas nor a liquid but possesses properties of both. The critical state of carbon dioxide is established by the phase diagram in **Figure 2**; varying the temperature and pressure changes the phase from solid to liquid to gas. However, at the critical point (the intersection of Tc and Pc), the difference between the liquid and gas phases disappears. The single fluid phase of carbon dioxide at this point is supposed to be "supercritical". The decellularization of mammalian tissues was successfully carried out using the extractive properties of $SCCO_2$ technology (**Figure 3**). To eliminate the immunogenicity of xenogeneic and allogeneic tissues requires decellularization. The decellularization process of the tissues to ECM scaffolds is to remove cells and antigens from the source tissue material. The ECM scaffold developed as an outcome of the decellularization process is the ECM consisting of proteins such as collagen, laminin, elastin, proteoglycans, and glycoproteins, as well as essential growth factors, angiogenesis factors [24]. Many porcine tissues and organs had been decellularized by the $SCCO_2$ process (**Figures 3** and **4**) and had been applied in several different medical applications by our team as listed in **Table 5**.

6.1 Aorta

The first effort for the decellularization of the porcine aorta employing $SCCO_2$ with the cosolvent as absolute ethanol was reported in 2008 [42]. The structural

Decellularization procedures	Tissues and organs
Supercritical carbon dioxide extraction technology	Bone, skin, cornea, cartilage, nerve, tendons, artery, pericardium, aortic-pulmonary valve, heart, liver, kidney, pancreas
Non-ionic detergents (Triton X-100)	Subcutaneous adipose tissue, myocardium, pericardium, aortic-pulmonary valve, gingiva, dental pulp, bone, skin, cornea, cartilage, artery, tendon, liver, kidney, pancreas
Ionic detergents (sodium dodecyl sulphate (SDS))	Muscle, tendons, adipose tissue, heart, pericardium, valves, artery, liver, kidney, testis, ovary, placentam, cornea
Zwitterionic detergents (CHAPS)	Arteries, lung, heart, esophagus, cornea, nerve, liver
Sonication	Cartilage, kidney, artery, larynx, meniscus, trachea, aorta, nerve, cornea, osteochondral tissue, meniscus, intervertebral disc, adipose tissue, heart
High-pressure gradient system	Artery, soft tissue, heart tissue, cornea, aorta, kidney, pericardium, bone matrix
Enzymes	Cornea, amniotic membrane, pancreas, tracheal cartilage, atery, dermis, tendon, larynx, nerve, heart values, umblical cord artery, amniotic membrane, aorta, muscle
Solvents	Cornea, placenta, kidney, liver, dental pulp, heart, dermis

Table 4.
Decellularization techniques are used for tissues and organs.

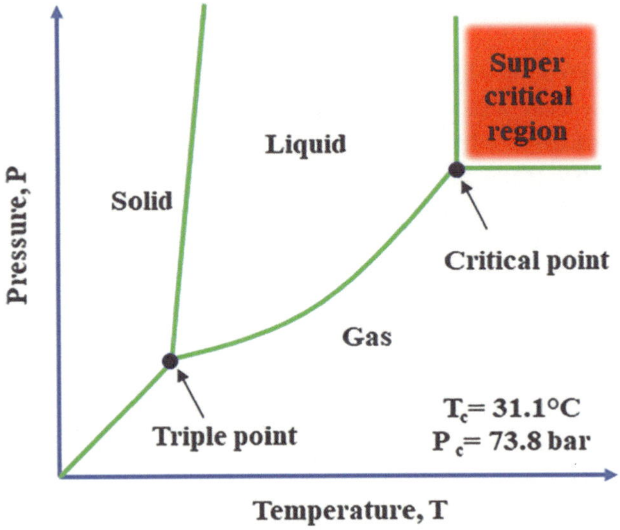

Figure 2.
Phase diagram of CO_2.

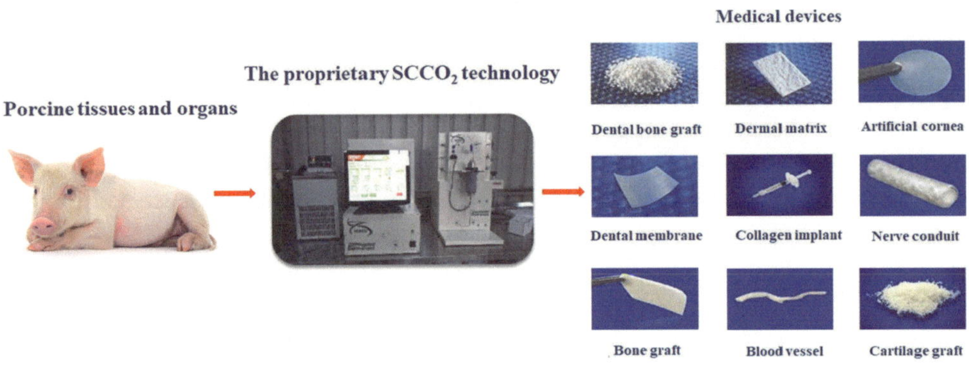

Figure 3.
Production of collagen scaffolds by $SCCO_2$ technology.

analysis depicted that the addition of ethanol encourages the removal of cellular material such as nuclei and phospholipids, which was unattainable without the use of $SCCO_2$ as a cosolvent. The results showed a decrease in the amount of phospholipids which depends on the time of processing, pressure, and rate of venting in the reactor. Altering the conditions, the lowest residual amount of phospholipids was 20%, which was attained as a result of 20 min at 15 MPa and 37°C. During the progression $SCCO_2$ process with the ethanol system, the aorta obtains rigidity, which reflects upon the character of the stress-strain diagrams. It is related to the dehydration of the aorta tissue due to the hygroscopic nature of ethanol and $SCCO_2$ dissolves up to 0.5% water [43]. The insignificant changes in mechanical properties and the deviations are not functionally significant [42]. This is the basics in the field of $SCCO_2$ decellularization; however, this process was not continued, due to the fast progress of methods of decellularization using detergents, enzymes, and other physicochemical methods. The preparation of biomaterials using $SCCO_2$ was resumed due to renovating the interest

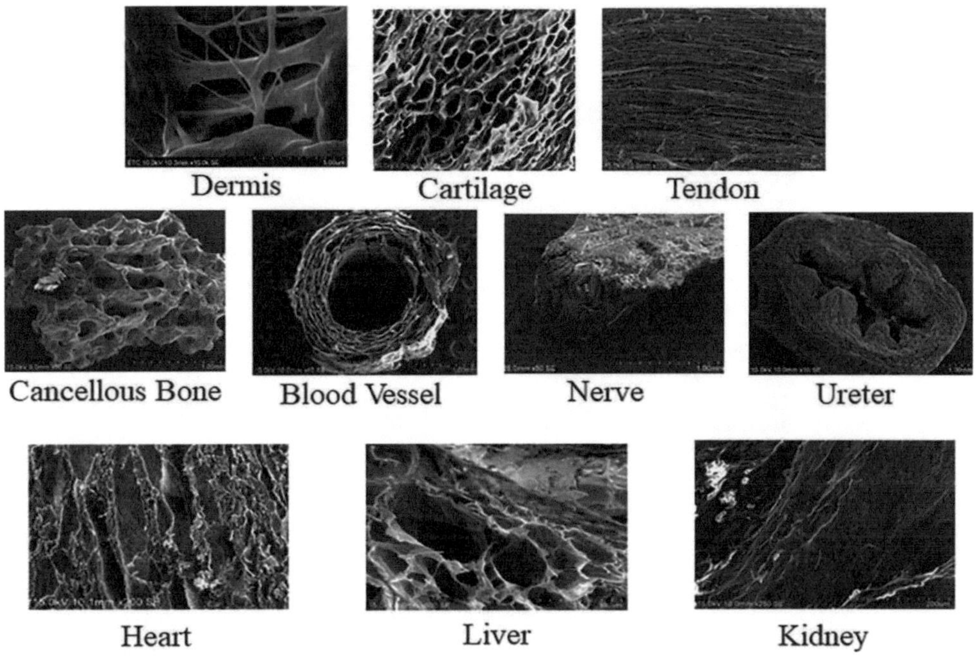

Figure 4.
Natural collagen scaffolds prepared by $SCCO_2$ technology.

Supercritical carbon dioxide extraction technology	
Princple	The carbon dioxide gas above a critical temperature, Tc = 31.1°C and pressure, Pc = 73.8 bar is said to be supercritical. In this state, carbon dioxide is neither a gas nor a liquid but possess properties of both. At the critical point, the difference between the liquid and gas phases disappears. The single fluid phase of carbon dioxide at this point is supposed to be 'supercritical'. This supercritical liquid can penetrate the tissue and organs efficiently to break down cellular components, which are washed off, with unaltered ECM scaffold.
Advantages	Green technology, cost-effectively, low temperatures, non-flammable, easily available, non-toxic, non-explosive, no chemical traces, no organic solvent, low viscosity, low surface tension, high density, gentle treatment, high productivity, fast and efficient, continuous and automatic with very low idle and turnaround time, non-corrosive, odorless, colorless. "Generally Regarded as Safe".
Disadvantages	No known disadvantages related to tissue decellularization. However, expensive equipment and the analysis process. Operated at the high pressure 1000–5000 psi.
Applications	Organ snd tissue decellularization, which can be used as a "high end medical devises".

Table 5.
Supercritical carbon dioxides principle, advantages, disadvantages and applications.

in solving the problems of decellularization and the factors such as the growth of new instrumentation, transition to green chemistry.

In the $SCCO_2$ decellularization process, the native collagen scaffold remains completely intact, even the smallest of the collagen strand (**Figure 5**, dermis ECM) as shown in the scanning electron microscopic photos of several different porcine tissues and organs. Therefore, we believe $SCCO_2$ decellularization is superior to other decellularization processes and thus the holy grail technology for the preparation of

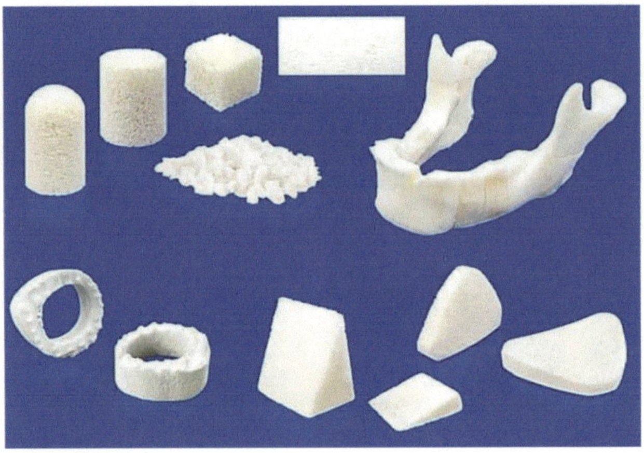

Figure 5.
Porcine bone derived products.

collagen scaffolds for tissue engineering and regenerative medicine. The process of decellularization of the aorta by $SCCO_2$ was continued in 2017 by altering the protocol using 70% ethanol and the processing was executed for 1 h at 37°C in addition 17.2 and 31 Mpa [44]. The results of histological studies and residual DNA exhibited complete elimination of the cellular debris from the aorta tissue is accomplished at 31 MPa. However, the ECM structure of the aorta is significantly altered at higher pressure, and the organization of the layers of the aorta external and internal layers is altered. These alterations in the aorta are capable of encouraging the development of embolism and aneurism in the case of grafting, which is a severe constraint for the clinical use of the aorta graft. In addition, these alterations of the aorta structure change the mechanical properties of an ECM.

To treat ischemic diseases, cardiac tissues were decellularized using $SCCO_2$with a cosolvent of absolute ethanol, leading to the formation of a hydrogel-based on an ECM, a source of glycosaminoglycans, proteins, and growth factors [26]. To attain the determined effect, the pressure was elevated to 35 MPa, and the time of the processing was extended to 6 h. The cardiac tissues were then rinsed in a solution of DNase I for 5 days. ECM components responsible for angiogenesis are preserved in the $SCCO_2$ decellularization; however, 1% SDS altered the ECM. Upon subcutaneous implantation of the hydrogel to mice induced angiogenesis. Subsequently encouraged the development of vessels to a significantly superior extent in comparison with the SDS treated and control gel based on type I collagen. Therefore, decellularization using the $SCCO_2$ opens up projections for the progression of bioinks for bioprinters and the formation of three-dimensional structures based on hydrogels [26].

6.2 Cornea

The porcine cornea was decellularized by $SCCO_2$ [45], the cornea tissue was initially subjected to osmotic shock by changing 2 M NaCl solution and deionized water. The process of $SCCO_2$ was done with the cosolvent addition of 60% ethanol at 35 MPa and 45°C for 80 min. In this process, it is likely to eliminate cellular components from the corneal tissue with the conservation of the suitable optical properties of the cornea. However, the decrease in the quantity of glycosaminoglycans and structural proteins during the processing in $SCCO_2$ directed to the alterations of the structural organization of the corneal ECM. In the traditional procedure decellularization by Triton X-100, the effect was less noticeable. The transplantation of the $SCCO_2$ decellularized cornea to rabbits showed regeneration of the cornea in 2 months, which confirmed the migration of keratocytes and corneal epithelial cells to the implanted cornea. In addition, no adverse rejections, inflammation, or angiopoiesis was observed in the implanted cornea. For the first time, the results of the regeneration of corneal tissues with the use of $SCCO_2$ decellularized transplants over the long term were described. The physical decellularization method of the cornea was established previously by the destruction of cells under the action of high pressure up to 100 MPa. However, the high-pressure method involves complex and costly hardware.

The $SCCO_2$-decellularized corneas displayed intact stromal structures and appropriate mechanical properties and had biocompatibility. Additionally, no immunological reactions and neovascularization were observed after lamellar keratoplasty in rabbits without complications. The transplanted decellularized corneas became transparent within 2 weeks of surgery. The decellularized corneas were completely re-epithelialized within 4 weeks. In conclusion, $SCCO_2$ decellularized corneas could be an ideal and useful scaffold for corneal tissue engineering [16]. The $SCCO_2$ technology-mediated production of the acellular porcine cornea (APC) depicted complete cells and non-collagenous protein removal relative to the Triton-sodium dodecyl sulfate decellularization process. APC presented excellent biocompatibility in rabbit lamellar corneal transplantation with a follow-up to 1 year. APC can be a potential substitute for human-donated cornea for corneal transplantation in the near future [18].

6.3 Bone

Decellularized bone tissue matrix produced by $SCCO_2$ [46], bovine cancellous bone was treated at 35 MPa and 50°C for 30 min with 25 min in a dynamic mode at a rate of the flow of $SCCO_2$ of 16.9 g/min and 5 min in a static mode of supercritical process. Subsequently, bovine cancellous bone was treated with a 7% solution of NaCl for 12 h first and then in a 0.1% solution of H_2O_2 for 48 h. On comparing lipid removal in bovine cancellous bone by $SCCO_2$ with traditional extraction with n-hexane in a Soxhlet apparatus, the $SCCO_2$ removed lipids 14% more efficiently. The biocompatibility of the $SCCO_2$ decellularized bone was proved by seeding and culturing with mesenchymal stem cells. However, mechanical properties and immunogenicity of the $SCCO_2$ decellularized bone were not determined. Similarly, xenogeneic bone decellularization [47] by $SCCO_2$ was done by rinsing with a 3% H_2O_2 solution and processing in the subcritical water, and final processing in $SCCO_2$.

The $SCCO_2$ technology was used to produce a series of novel decellularized porcine collagen bone grafts (DPB) in an assortment of shapes and sizes (**Figure 5**, cancellous bone). The native intact collagen was preserved in the $SCCO_2$ processed DPB was confirmed by Masson trichrome staining. The cytotoxicity and biocompatibility tests according to ISO10993 and their efficacy for bone regeneration in osteochondral defects in rabbits were evaluated. The rabbit pyrogen test confirmed DPB was non-toxic. *In vitro* and *in vivo* biocompatibility tests of the DPB did not show any toxic or mutagenic effects. *in vitro* cytotoxicity test, *in vivo* pyrogen study, *in vitro* mammalian cell gene mutation test, and systemic toxicity study in SD rats. The DPB produced by $SCCO_2$ exhibited similar chemical characteristics to human bone, no toxicity, good biocompatibility, and enhanced bone regeneration in rabbits. Therefore, the potential application of the $SCCO_2$ extraction technique to generate a native decellularized bone scaffold for regeneration in human clinical trials [10]. The DPB produced by $SCCO_2$ on alveolar socket healing after tooth extraction had promising bone regeneration properties similar to that of Bio-Oss® in a canine tooth extraction socket model [15].

The DPB produced by $SCCO_2$ ABCcolla® Collagen Bone Graft, was used for the reconstruction of the orbital framework in humans. The orbital defects were fixed by the implantation of the ABCcolla® Collagen Bone Graft. All subjects showed improvement of enophthalmos on computerized tomography at week 8 follow-up. No replacement of implants was needed during follow-ups. Thus, ABCcolla® Collagen Bone Graft proved to be safe and effective in the reconstruction of the orbital floor with high accessibility, high stability, good biocompatibility, low infection rate, and low complication rate [17]. The DPB produced by $SCCO_2$ seeded with adipose-derived stem cells (ASCs) boosted callus formation in a segmental femoral defect. The mechanism of DPB might be modulation in the expression of BMP 2 and osteocalcin, thus leading to enhanced bone regeneration and new bone formation in a rat segmental femoral defect model. Thus the DPB scaffold is an excellent biomaterial for bone tissue repair. Implantation of the DPB seeded ASCs stimulated endochondral ossification for substantial bone regeneration. The DPB seeded ASCs system is of clinical relevance for segmental defect bone regeneration [19].

6.4 Acellular dermal matrix

The $SCCO_2$ decellularized porcine acellular dermal matrix (ADM) seeded with autologous adipose-derived stem cells (ASCs) in streptozotocin (STZ)-induced diabetes mellitus rats showed the wound healing rate increased in diabetes mellitus. Diabetes mellitus wound treated with ADM-ASCs showed a significantly higher wound healing. ADM-ASC-treated rats showed significantly increased epidermal growth factor, Ki67, and prolyl 4-hydroxylase and significantly decreased CD45. The intervention comprising ADM decellularized from porcine skin by using $SCCO_2$ and ASCs was proven to improve diabetic wound healing. The $SCCO_2$ produced ADM-ASCs had a positive effect on epidermal regeneration, anti-inflammation, collagen production and processing, and cell proliferation; thus, it accelerated wound healing [14].

6.5 Cartilage

Cartilage tissue engineering that combines the triads of decellularized porcine cartilage graft as a scaffold, plasma rich platelet (PRP) as signal, and chondrocytes as the cell to attenuate anterior cruciate ligament transection (ACLT)-induced OA progression and regenerate the knee cartilage in rats. The $SCCO_2$ decellularized porcine cartilage graft (dPCG) significantly reduced the ACLT-induced OA symptoms and attenuated the OA progression. The histological analysis depicted cartilage protection by dPCG. The repair and attenuation effect were proved by dPCG in the articular knee cartilage damage as evidenced by safranin-O, type II collagen, aggrecan, and SOX-9 immuno-staining. To conclude, intra-articular administration of dPCG with or without PRP is efficient in repairing the damaged cartilage in the experimental OA model [21]. A 3D composite was constructed using $SCCO_2$-dPCG that promotes chondrogenic marker expression *in vitro*. The *in vivo* implantation of 3D composite to cartilage defect exhibited significant regeneration by increasing the expression of Collagen type II and aggrecan. The bioengineered 3D composite by combining dPCG scaffold, chondrocytes, and PRP facilitated the chondrogenic marker expression in both *in vitro* and *in vivo* models with accelerated cartilage regeneration. This might serve the purpose of clinical treatment of large focal articular cartilage defects in humans in the near future [22].

6.6 Nasal cartilage

A bioactive 3D histotypic $SCCO_2$ decellularized nasal cartilage (dPNCG) construct was engineered with adipose-derived stem cells (ADSC) and chondrocytes and cultured for 21 days. The 3D histotypic constructs produced a solid mass of 3D histotypic cartilage with significant production of glycosaminoglycans. The $SCCO_2$-dPNCG granules are bound to one another by extracellular matrix and proteoglycan, to form a 3D structure expressed chondrogenic markers such, as type II collagen, aggrecan, and SOX-9. The $SCCO_2$-dPNCG substrate enabled the synthesis of type II collagen along with ECM to yield 3D histotypic cartilage. This engineered 3D construct might serve as a promising future candidate for cartilage tissue engineering in rhinoplasty [20].

6.7 Atelocollagen

Atelocollagen was prepared by using $SCCO_2$ technology. To our knowledge, we are the first to use $SCCO_2$ technology to produce atelocollagen. The sliced porcine skin was subjected to a proprietary $SCCO_2$ for decellularization. The decellularized porcine skin scaffold was freeze-dried and freeze-milled to granules and subjected to enzymatic hydrolysis using pepsin in acidic conditions, then subjected to ultrafiltration for pepsin and telopeptide removal. The atelocollagen solution was filtered through a 0.2-μm filter for sterilization. The acidic atelocollagen solution was subjected to fibrillogenesis by bringing the pH to 7, then centrifuged to obtain the atelocollagen slurry. This slurry was then freeze-dried to obtain atelocollagen dry powder [12]. The whole process saves a lot of time and cost as compared to the traditional collagen purification process. Atelocollagen prepared by $SCCO_2$ followed by pepsin digestion of the telo-peptides process showed complete removal of the telo-peptides as compared to the traditional purification process [12].

6.8 Skin

The $SCCO_2$ technology was employed to decellularize porcine skin to produce a collagen matrix (**Figure 6**). This novel collagen matrix was developed to accelerate wound healing for hard-to-heal or delayed wound healing clinical conditions. The collagen matrix produced by $SCCO_2$ technology from porcine skin is chemically comparable and biocompatible to human skin. The $SCCO_2$ produced collagen matrix showed complete decellularization, the chemical content was found to be type I collagen and characteristic features were similar to that of humans. The collagen matrix proved to be non-toxic in *in vitro* cytotoxicity-agar diffusion test, *in vivo* pyrogen study, *in vitro* mammalian cell gene mutation test, acute systemic toxicity study in mice, systemic toxicity study in SD rats, intracutaneous irritation test, skin sensitization study (maximization test), and muscle implant study. In the porcine excision full-thickness skin wound healing model, the collagen matrix cocultured with fibroblast and keratinocytes exhibited decreased inflammation, complete epithelization, and enhanced wound healing [11].

6.9 Adipose tissue

The $SCCO_2$ process was used for the decellularization of adipose tissue extracellular matrix [48]. The adipose tissue was subjected to the $SCCO_2$ process for 3 h at 18 MPa and 37°C with the addition of ethanol as the cosolvent. The decellularized adipose

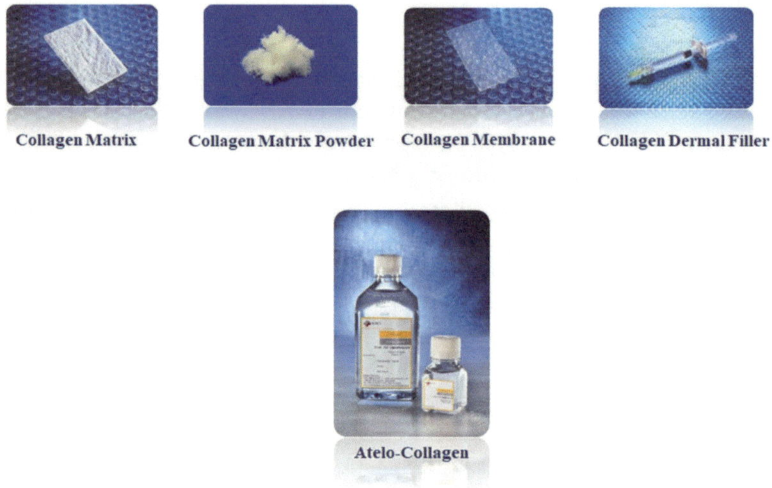

Figure 6.
Porcine skin derived products.

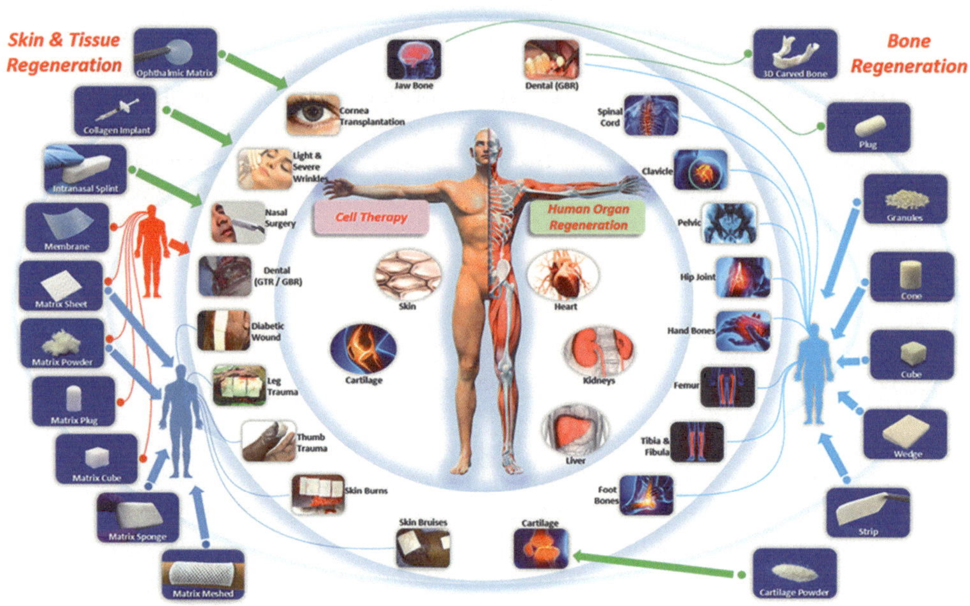

Figure 7.
$SCCO_2$ decellularized biomaterials for TERM.

tissue consisted of the extracellular matrix components and was free from lipids. The decellularized adipose tissue extracellular matrix can help the widespread coating progress the adhesion of cells due to the presence of active components such as collagen, laminin, elastin, fibronectin, and glycosaminoglycans. The coating of the decellularized adipose tissue extracellular matrix increases the proliferation of human endothelial cells isolated from umbilical vein, human adipose tissue-derived mesenchymal stem cells, human monocytic leukemia cells, and immortalized human keratinocytes on a plastic culture plate and does not induce the production of the proinflammatory phenotype of macrophages. The decellularized adipose tissue extracellular matrix was used as a model for the investigation of the action of anticancer drugs on cells for breast cancer, which is similar to the native condition [49]. The $SCCO_2$ decellularization contrasts with the prevailing methods in the rapidity and cost-effective nature. Traditional methods of decellularization of adipose tissue include several freezing-thawing cycles, extraction of lipids with isopropanol, and enzymatic treatment [49, 50]. The development of the $SCCO_2$ decellularization for the preparation of an extracellular matrix from adipose tissue is an environmentally friendly approach that will endorse the development of the methods of tissue engineering with the use of autologous material.

We produce tissue and organ scaffold using $SCCO_2$ extraction technology, such as liver, kidney, heart, pancreas, artery, skin, bone, cartilage, and cornea [13]. **Table 5** listed our works on the various tissue and organ scaffolds extracted by $SCCO_2$ technology for tissue engineering applications [13]. The ultimate goal of TERM is to use the tissues and organs produced by $SCCO_2$ from the porcine or bovine to regenerate the human tissues and organs (**Figure 7**). We hope to develop the whole animal application without any waste materials, which suits the purpose of the circular economy. Eventually, we intend to regenerate any human tissue and organ by its animal counterpart.

7. Conclusions

Substantial progression in the field of TERM and scaffold biomaterials engineering by $SCCO_2$ proposes extended potentials to acquire novel, effective achievements, which may be applied in biomedical applications. Recently, the interest in natural biomaterials produced by $SCCO_2$ technology for medical devices production has increased, and a greater number of in-depth studies are done to better detect their likely applications related to chemical and physical characteristics and the extraction procedures, which do not modify their structural properties and biocompatibility. Tissue engineering approaches have become a valid alternative for body structure and function restoring, natural scaffold biomaterials produced by $SCCO_2$ technology are also used as biomimetic scaffolds with controlled degradation rate *in vivo* and regeneration. *In vitro* and *in vivo* studies have shown the advantages related to natural scaffold biomaterials produced by $SCCO_2$ technology use in the regenerative medicine field.

The $SCCO_2$ decellularization technology as compared to other traditional processes is a minimally manipulated process and thus cost-effective, and gentle to the natural collagen scaffold ECM structure. Therefore, $SCCO_2$ decellularized scaffolds might contain unaltered signals that are indispensable for stem cell adhesion, migration, homing, proliferation, and differentiation. No chemicals and solvents were involved in the process, therefore it is eco-friendly. It destroys bacteria and inactivates viruses during the process. $SCCO_2$ technology costs only about 1/10th of the traditional process. Different tissues and organs from animals such as pigs, cows, horses, sheep can be used to produce decellularized scaffolds. The most important and key point is $SCCO_2$ process drastically reduces immune rejection.

Our study indicated that the natural collagen scaffolds prepared by the $SCCO_2$ process might be able to induce stem cell differentiation *in vivo*, with the help of the growth factors and cytokines in the microenvironment. The signal for stem cell differentiation could be pre-built by the combination of various genotypes of 29 collagen polypeptides during scaffold synthesis, which exhibits different signals in different tissues and organs that guide the stem cells to differentiate into the right cell types.

The revelation of this intrinsic signal will be our future research focus. Before that, we boldly hypothesize that any organ decellularized by the $SCCO_2$, with the intact scaffold structure, can be reconstructed *in vivo* when implanted back into the live animal with the proper connection of blood circulation to bring in the stem cells required for the organ regeneration. We are testing this hypothesis and hope to find out soon. The application of biomaterials produced by $SCCO_2$ technology to tissue engineering, in modern-day science is using the natural biomaterial with the most suitable performance *in vivo*, able to promote cell proliferation and differentiation in damaged tissue to restore the normal architecture of ECM. To conclude, TERM strategies particularly in the orthopedic and plastic surgery clinical field epitomize an effective and sophisticated alternative for the future, but their success firmly rests on an ever in-depth knowledge regarding the features of the scaffold biomaterial.

Acknowledgements

This research was financially supported by the Southern Taiwan Science Park Bureau, (107SMIC-RC02; BX-01-03-05-108 and 108CB01), Taiwan, R.O.C.

Author details

Periasamy Srinivasan and Dar-Jen Hsieh*
R&D Center, ACRO Biomedical Co., Ltd., Kaohsiung City, Taiwan

*Address all correspondence to: dj@acrobimomedical.com

References

[1] Langer R, Vacanti JP. Tissue engineering. Science. 1993; **260**(5110):920-926

[2] Han F, Wang J, Ding L, Hu Y, Li W, Yuan Z, et al. Tissue engineering and regenerative medicine: Achievements, future, and sustainability in Asia. Frontiers in Bioengineering and Biotechnology. 2020;**8**:83

[3] Salgado AJ, Oliveira JM, Martins A, Teixeira FG, Silva NA, Neves NM, et al. Tissue engineering and regenerative medicine: Past, present, and future. International Review of Neurobiology. 2013;**108**:1-33

[4] Frey BM, Zeisberger SM, Hoerstrup SP. Tissue engineering and regenerative medicine—new initiatives for individual treatment offers. Transfusion Medicine and Hemotherapy. 2016;**43**:318-319

[5] Goldstein SA, Moalli MR. Current concepts in tissue engineering: Cell, matrices, and genes. Current Opinion in Orthopaedics. 2001;**12**(5):424-427

[6] Alberts B, Johnson A, Lewis J, Raff M, Roberts K. Molecular Biology of the Cell. New York, NY, USA: Garland Science; 2002

[7] Parenteau-Bareil R, Gauvin R, Berthod F. Collagen-based biomaterials for tissue engineering applications. Materials (Basel). 2010;**3**(3):1863-1887

[8] Badylak SF, Gilbert TW. Immune response to biologic scaffold materials. Seminars in Immunology. 2008;**20**(2):109-116

[9] Veryasova NN, Lazhko AE, Isaev DE, Grebenik EA, Timashev PS. Supercritical carbon dioxide—a powerful tool for green biomaterial chemistry. Russian Journal of Physical Chemistry B. 2019;**13**:1079-1087

[10] Chen YW, Hsieh DJ, Periasamy S, Yen KC, Wang HC, Chien HH. Development of a decellularized porcine bone graft by supercritical carbon dioxide extraction technology for bone regeneration. Journal of Tissue Engineering and Regenerative Medicine. 2021;**15**(4):401-414

[11] Wang CH, Hsieh DJ, Periasamy S, Chuang CT, Tseng FW, Kuo JC, et al. Regenerative porcine dermal collagen matrix developed by supercritical carbon dioxide extraction technology: Role in accelerated wound healing. Materialia. 2020;**9**:100576

[12] Hsieh DJ, Srinivasan P. Protocols for accelerated production and purification of collagen scaffold and atelocollagen from animal tissues. BioTechniques. 2020;**69**(3):220-225

[13] Hsieh DJ, Srinivasan P, Yen KC, Yeh YC, Chen YJ, Wang HC, et al. Protocols for the preparation and characterization of decellularized tissue and organ scaffolds for tissue engineering. BioTechniques. 2021;**70**(2):107-115

[14] Chou PR, Lin YN, Wu SH, Lin SD, Srinivasan P, Hsieh DJ, et al. Supercritical carbon dioxide-decellularized porcine acellular dermal matrix combined with autologous adipose-derived stem cells: Its role in accelerated diabetic wound healing. International Journal of Medical Sciences. 2020;**17**(3):354-367

[15] Chen YW, Chen MY, Hsieh DJ, Periasamy S, Yen KC, Chuang CT,

et al. Evaluating the bone-regenerative role of the decellularized porcine bone xenograft in a canine extraction socket model. Clinical and Experimental Dental Research. 2021;**7**(4):409-418

[16] Huang YH, Tseng FW, Chang WH, Peng IC, Hsieh DJ, Wu SW, et al. Preparation of acellular scaffold for corneal tissue engineering by supercritical carbon dioxide extraction technology. Acta Biomaterialia. 2017;**58**:238-243

[17] Huang CH, Hsieh DJ, Wu YC, Yen KC, Srinivasan P, Lee HC, et al. Reconstruction of the orbital floor using supercritical CO_2 decellularized porcine bone graft. International Journal of Medical Sciences. 2021;**18**(16):3684-3691

[18] Liang CM, Hsieh DJ, Tseng FW, Srinivasan P, Yeh ML, Tai MC. Acellular porcine cornea produced by supercritical carbon dioxide extraction: A potential substitute for human corneal regeneration. Cornea. 2021. DOI: 10.1097/ICO.0000000000002790. Online ahead of print

[19] Liu K-F, Chen R-F, Li Y-T, Lin Y-N, Hsieh D-J, Periasamy S, et al. Supercritical carbon dioxide decellularized bone matrix seeded with adipose-derived mesenchymal stem cells accelerated bone regeneration. Biomedicine. 2021;**9**(12):1825

[20] Lee SS, Wu YC, Huang SH, Chen YC, Srinivasan P, Hsieh DJ, et al. A novel 3D histotypic cartilage construct engineered by supercritical carbon dioxide decellularized porcine nasal cartilage graft and chondrocytes exhibited chondrogenic capability in vitro. International Journal of Medical Sciences. 2021;**18**(10):2217-2227

[21] Wu CC, Tarng YW, Hsu DZ, Srinivasan P, Yeh YC, Lai YP, et al. Supercritical carbon dioxide decellularized porcine cartilage graft with PRP attenuated OA progression and regenerated articular cartilage in ACLT-induced OA rats. Journal of Tissue Engineering and Regenerative Medicine. 2021;**15**:1118-1130. DOI: 10.1002/term.3252. Online ahead of print

[22] Chen YT, Lee HS, Hsieh DJ, Periasamy S, Yeh YC, Lai YP, et al. 3D composite engineered using supercritical CO_2 decellularized porcine cartilage scaffold, chondrocytes, and PRP: Role in articular cartilage regeneration. Journal of Tissue Engineering and Regenerative Medicine. 2021;**15**(2):163-175

[23] Crapo P, Gilbert T, Badylak S. An overview of tissue and whole organ decellularization processes. Biomaterials. 2011;**32**:3233-3243

[24] Petersen TH, Calle EA, Zhao L, Lee EJ, Gui L, Raredon MB, et al. Tissue-engineered lungs for in vivo implantation. Science. 2010;**329**:538-541

[25] Choi JS, Kim BS, Kim JY, Kim JD, Choi YC, Yang HJ, et al. Decellularized extracellular matrix derived from human adipose tissue as a potential scaffold for allograft tissue engineering. Journal of Biomedical Materials Research Part A. 2011;**97A**:292-299

[26] Seo Y, Jung Y, Kim SH. Decellularized heart ECM hydrogel using supercritical carbon dioxide for improved angiogenesis. Acta Biomaterialia. 2017;**67**:2708-2281

[27] Hwang J, San BH, Turner NJ, White LJ, Faulk DM, Badylak SF, et al. Molecular assessment of collagen denaturation in decellularized tissues using collagen hybridizing peptide. Acta Biomaterialia. 2017;**53**:268-278

[28] Reing JE, Brown BN, Daly KA, Freund JM, Gilbert TW, Hsiong SX,

et al. The effects of processing methods upon mechanical and biologic properties of porcine dermal extracellular matrix scaffolds. Biomaterials. 2010;**31**: 8626-8633

[29] Mendoza-novelo B, Castellano LE, Padilla-miranda RG, Lona-ramos MC, Cuéllar-mata P, Vega-gonzález A, et al. The component leaching from decellularized pericardial bioscaffolds and its implication in the macrophage response: Decellularized Pericardial Bioscaffolds. Journal of Biomedical Materials Research Part A. 2016;**104**:2810-2822

[30] Sun WQ, Xu H, Sandor M, Lombardi J. Process-induced extracellular matrix alterations affect the mechanisms of soft tissue repair and regeneration. Journal of Tissue Engineering. 2013;**4**:2041731413505305

[31] Mendoza-novelo B, Avila EE, Cauich-rodríguez JV, Jorge-herrero E, Rojo FJ, Guinea GV, et al. Decellularization of pericardial tissue and its impact on tensile viscoelasticity and glycosaminoglycan content. Acta Biomaterialia. 2011;**7**:1241-1248

[32] Oryan A, Alidadi S, Moshiri A, Maffulli N. Bone regenerative medicine: Classic options, novel strategies, and future directions. Journal of Orthopaedic Surgery and Research. 2014;**9**(1):18

[33] Chappard D, Fressonnet C, Genty C, Baslé MF, Rebel A. Fat in bone xenografts: Importance of the purification procedures on cleanliness, wettability and biocompatibility. Biomaterials. 1993;**14**:507-512

[34] Gardin C, Ricci S, Ferroni L, Guazzo R, Sbricoli L, De Benedictis G, et al. Decellurisation and delipidation protocols of bovine bone and pericardium for bone grafting and guided bone regeneration procedures. PLoS One. 2015;**10**(7):e0132344

[35] Ghassemi T, Saghatoleslami N, Mahdavi-Shahri N, Matin MM, Gheshlaghi R, Moradi A. A comparison study of different decellularization treatments on bovine articular cartilage. Journal of Tissue Engineering and Regenerative Medicine. 2019; **13**(10):1861-1871

[36] Graham ME, Gratzer PF, Bezuhly M, Hong P. Development and characterization of decellularized human nasoseptal cartilage matrix for use in tissue engineering. The Laryngoscope. 2016;**126**:2226-2231

[37] Elder BD, Kim DH, Athanasiou KA. Developing an articular cartilage decellularization process toward facet joint cartilage replacement. Neurosurgery. 2010;**66**(4):722-727

[38] Luo Z, Bian Y, Su W, Shi L, Li S, Song Y, et al. Comparison of various reagents for preparing a decellularized porcine cartilage scaffold. American Journal of Translational Research. 2019;**11**(3):1417-1427

[39] Bautista CA, Park HJ, Mazur CM, Aaron RK, Bilgen B. Effects of chondroitinaseabc-mediatedproteoglycan digestion on decellularization and recellularization of articular cartilage. PLoS One. 2016;**11**(7):e0158976

[40] Vashi AV, Werkmeister JA, Vuocolo T, Elvin CM, Ramshaw JA. Stabilization of collagen tissues by photocrosslinking. Journal of Biomedical Materials Research Part A. 2012;**100**:2239-2243

[41] Bernhardt A, Wehrl M, Paul V, Hochmuth T, Schumacher M, Schutz K, et al. Improved sterilization of sensitive biomaterials with supercritical carbon

dioxide at low temperature. PLoS One. 2015;**10**:e0129205

[42] Sawada K, Terada D, Yamaoka T, Kitamura S, Fujisato T. Cell removal with supercritical carbon dioxide for acellular artificial tissue. Journal of Chemical Technology & Biotechnology. 2008;**83**:943-949

[43] Sabirzyanov N, Win A, Akhunov A, Gumerov A. Solubility of water in supercritical carbon dioxide. High Temperature. 2002;**40**:203-206

[44] Guler S, Asian V, Hosseinian P, Aydin H, et al. Tissue Engineering Methods (Part C). 2017;**23**:540-547

[45] Hashimoto Y, Funamoto S, Sasaki S, Honda T, Hattori S, Nam K, et al. Preparation and characterization of decellularized cornea using high-hydrostatic pressurization for corneal tissue engineering. Biomaterials. 2010;**31**:3941-3948

[46] Smolentsev DV, Gurin MV, Venediktov AA, Evdokimov SV, Fadeev RA. Purification of xenogeneic bone matrix by extraction with supercritical carbon dioxide and evaluation of the obtained material. Russian Journal of Physical Chemistry B. 2017;**11**:1283-1287

[47] Zalepugin DY, Zaitzev VV, Tilkunova NA, Chernyshova IV, Selezneva II, Nikonova YA, et al. Xenogenic bone matrix treated with supercritical carbon dioxide as a potential osteoplastic material. Russian Journal of Physical Chemistry B. 2015;**9**:1005-1010

[48] Wang JK, Luo B, Guneta V, Li L, Foo SEM, Dai Y, et al. Supercritical carbon dioxide extracted extracellular matrix material from adipose tissue. Materials Science and Engineering C. 2017;**75**:349-358

[49] Flynn L. The use of decellularized adipose tissue to provide an inductive microenvironment for the adipogenic differentiation of human adipose-derived stem cells. Biomaterials. 2010;**31**:4715-4724

[50] Brown V, Freund J, Han L, Rubin J, Reing J, Jeffries E, et al. Comparison of three methods for the derivation of a biologic scaffold composed of adipose tissue extracellular matrix. Tissue Engineering Methods (Part C). 2011;**17**:411-421

Chapter 3

Nanoparticle Based Collagen Biomaterials for Wound Healing

Kausalya Neelavara Makkithaya, Sharmila Nadumane, Guan-Yu Zhuo, Sanjiban Chakrabarty and Nirmal Mazumder

Abstract

Wounds and infections are extremely common cases that are dealt with in the medical field. Their effective and timely treatment ensures the overall well-being of patients in general. Current treatments include the use of collagen scaffolds and other biomaterials for tissue regeneration. Although the use of collagenous biomaterials has been tested, the incorporation of nanoparticles into these collagenous biomaterials is a fairly new field, whose possibilities are yet to be explored and discovered. The current chapter explores the applications of the amalgamation of collagenous biomaterials with nanoparticles, which themselves are known to be effective in the treatment and prevention of infections.

Keywords: wound healing, nanoparticles, nanotechnology, collagen, biomaterials

1. Introduction

An injury that occurs in a quick manner, which often leaves the skin torn, cut, or punctured, or wherein the skin or any other tissues of the body undergoes acute trauma resulting in a contusion, is defined as a 'wound'. This is when the body's repair mechanism works to repair the damage by replacing the damaged tissue with newly synthesized tissue. This is characterized by a cascade of highly coordinated reactions that occur at the tissue damage region, working to restore normal tissue, which is called wound healing mechanism. This process requires nutrients and amino acids in adequate amounts to ensure the smooth repair of damaged cells, the supplementation of which has been viewed as a possible solution to augment the process and provide better strength and elasticity to the newly developing tissue [1].

It is known that collagen, being an integral part of most tissues in the body, plays an important role in the structural stability, elasticity, and tensile strength. It is therefore unsurprising that collagen is vital for restoring the structural integrity of the wounded tissue. It has been observed that, formation of scar tissue is an integral part of wound healing in most cases, with epidermal wounds being the exception. This scar tissue is composed primarily of collagen. This makes collagen synthesis an extremely crucial part of the wound healing process [2]. It is therefore practical to employ collagen supplements to augment and speed up the process of hound healing, and even enhance the tensile strength and other innate properties of the tissue. Through a study conducted by Felician et al., it was proven that collagen obtained from a species of jelly fish was indeed effective in escalating the pace of wound healing, making it a potential product that could be used in treating major wounds [3]. There is growing interest in the applications of collagen powder derived from marine sources to treat wounds effectively and reducing the possibility of a scar on the skin along with many other biomedical applications [4]. However, it must be understood that collagen powder is not the only form of collagen supplement for treatment of wounds and other tissue replacement procedures. There are a variety of forms, in which collagen is used as a biomaterial, for wound treatment [5].

Collagen derived from various sources is fabricated into various scaffolds, which can be implanted or grafted into the region of tissue damage, to act as an effective substrate for the attachment of precursor cells and allow their proliferation, thereby increasing the chances of tissue repair effectively. These precursor cells are multipotent adult stem cells which have the ability to differentiate to form various cells depending on the environment they are in, or the stimuli they receive for differentiation. These scaffolds can also be in the form of hydrogels, or fibers, and not just solid in nature. The use of collagen has proven to be effective for wound healing, due to the fact that it is an integral part of the extracellular matrix (ECM) on which most tissues are constructed [6]. Nanotechnology is a field of science that has been explored for its possible applications in the biomedical sector. Many nanomaterials such as nanoparticles and fibers are known to possess antimicrobial activities, which could be effective in the wound healing mechanism for the prevention of further infection. It is thereby prudent that the nanomaterials should be tried and tested along with those of collagen in order to come up with innovative methods to treat major wounds effectively. This chapter aims to summarize the importance of collagen and nanoparticles, synthesis of nano collagen in order to benefit from the wound healing properties of both nanoparticles and collagen, along with the areas of wound healing in which nano collagen is currently being used.

2. Nanotechnology

Nanotechnology is the branch of science and engineering that involves design, construction, and characterization of materials by restructuring the atoms and molecules with the size range of 1–100 nm in one or more dimensions [7, 8]. The engineered materials are nanomaterials that show distinct chemical and physical properties compared to the bulk materials due to the synthesis and assembly at the molecular level that can be exploited for commercial use [9]. Nanomaterials can be of different shapes mainly based on their dimensions i.e., nanoparticles of zero dimension, nanorods of one dimension, and nanosheets of two dimensions [10]. Nanoparticles, due to their small size have the ability to penetrate the bacterial cell wall, and though the cells metabolic pathway cause changes to the cell structure and function. Nanoparticles are also known to interact various components of the bacterial cell, such as lysosomes, enzymes, and ribosomes, thereby leading to oxidative stress, altered permeability of the cell membrane, protein deactivation, and altered gene expression, eventually causing cell death among the bacteria. Thus, it can be said that the Nanoparticles have antibacterial properties, which can be exploited for sterilization of larger wounds, thereby preventing infections from occurring during the wound healing process. When compared to the conventional wound healing drugs certain nanoparticles exhibit greater penetration of cell membrane [9]. Nanoparticles, nanocomposites, coatings, and scaffolds are the main nanomaterials used for wound healing (as shown in **Figure 1**). Nanoparticles can be (i) inorganic metal or non-metal (ii) organic non-polymeric or polymeric. Nanocomposites are made of porous materials, colloids, copolymers, or gels. Coating and scaffolds include hydrogels, nanofibers, films, and coatings [11]. Different classes of nanoparticles are involved for the treatment of wounds. They are discussed below:

2.1 Metallic nanoparticles

The antimicrobial property of metallic nanoparticles is exploited in wound management and can be used as a nanocarrier. The surface area to volume ratio of metallic nanoparticles is high. The small size enables them to cross barriers and penetrate the underlying layers of thick tissues like skin. These features make them ideal for drug delivery and to treat wounds. Some of the widely used metallic nanoparticles includes—silver nanoparticles (Ag NPs), gold nanoparticles (AuNPs), zinc oxide nanoparticles (ZnO NPs), iron oxide nanoparticles (IONPs), and titanium dioxide nanoparticles (TiO_2 NPs) [12].

2.2 Polymeric nanoparticles (PNPs)

Polymeric nanoparticles include polymer nanospheres and polymer nano capsules. Biologically active molecules such as drugs, genes, and fluorophores are absorbed on the surface of polymer nanospheres forming antibiotic incorporated nanoparticles (NPs). Griseofluvin (GF), one such NP, is known to function as an effective carrier of biologically active entities [12, 13]. The polymer nano capsules are vesicles where the core contains bioactive agents surrounded by polymeric shell. The polymers used in the preparation can be natural polymers like starch, polypeptides, albumin, sodium alginate, chitin, cellulose, gelatin, polyhydroxy alkanoates (PHAs) or artificial polymers like polyethylene glycol (PEG), poly lactic acid co-glycolic acid (PLGA), polyvinyl alcohol (PVA), polyvinyl pyrrolidone (PVP), polyethylene etc. They show higher encapsulation efficiency and high stability of encapsulated active substance that helps them in the effective delivery of drugs to targeted sites [13].

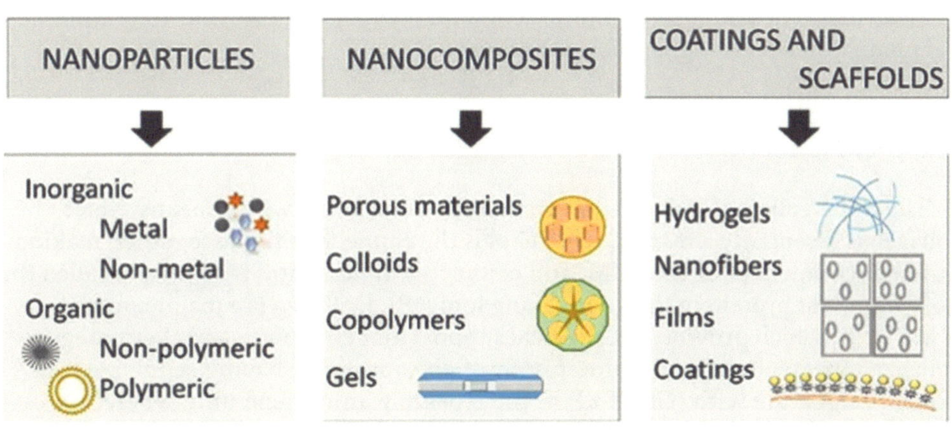

Figure 1.
Types of nanomaterials used for treatment of wounds. The figure is reproduced with permission from [11].

2.3 Nano emulsions

Nano emulsions shows small droplet size and high surface area that makes them a suitable vehicle for drug delivery to treat wounds. A unique feature of these nano emulsions is their ability to deliver hydrophobic drugs [14]. They also have long shelf life, and are easily formulated [12]. The components of nano emulsions include different oil types, emulsifying agents like sodium deoxycholate, sodium dodecyl sulphate, antioxidants, chelating agents, preservatives etc. [15].

2.4 Solid-lipid nanoparticles (SLNs)

Solid-lipid nanoparticles are used as drug vehicles in case of inflamed or damaged skin. They are efficient and non-toxic carriers of both lipophilic and hydrophilic drugs. The structure is made up of long-fatty acid chains of palmitic acid, stearic acid or arachidic acid taurocholate, emulsifiers, and water.

2.5 Nanofiber scaffolds/mats

Nanofiber scaffolds/mats, considered as a substitute to damaged ECM, are mainly used in the wound dressing due to its healing power and unique structure. As the scaffolds are applied on the wound there will be attachment of fibroblasts and formation of matrix that acts as ground substrate and aid in faster wound recovery. Manufacturing of nanofibrous scaffolds involves electrospinning that produces uniform nanofibers [16].

2.6 Nanogels

Hydrogels are used as delivery vehicles for wound treatment due to their properties such as high porosity which keeps the wound environment moist, and the presence of 3D polymeric matrix that absorbs the wound exudates allowing for proper permeation of oxygen [12]. While nanogels demonstrates some advanced features compared to those of hydrogels such as stability, ease of synthesis, quick response to stimulus, an adjustable size that can be exploited for drug delivery, controlled release of drugs, and tumor imaging. Nanogels are made up of chemical polymers and biomolecules. The nanogels of amino acids and polypeptides are easy to synthesize and modify and show higher biocompatibility [17].

3. Collagen

The word 'collagen' is derived from a Greek term 'kolla', which means 'Glue'. Collagen is essentially a matrix, which holds the connective tissue together, making it a major component of the ECM, and connective tissues, and is rightfully called the most abundant protein in the animal kingdom [18]. Collagen is a major component of the ECM, which provides mechanical support for cell growth and their integrity. Collagen represents an entire superfamily of glycoproteins, having, a polypeptide sequence signature with $[\text{Gly-X-Y}]_n$ as the repeating amino acid unit, wherein X and Y are proline and hydroxyproline respectively. Another salient feature of these glycoproteins is their noteworthy quaternary structure with the right-handed triple helix structure composed of three left-handed polyproline chains of uniform length.

The chains in the triple helix can either be identical, forming homotrimers as seen in collagen II, or be different from each other, forming heterotrimers, as seen in collagen IX. Presence of glycine is invariant in collagen and is known to stabilize the collagen structure. It has been found that the absence of glycine or any mutations to the same is known to cause disruption in the hydrogen bonds formed in collagen and distort the structure [19].

The presence of collagen and collagenous structures throughout the animal kingdom indicates its importance in biological structures. Collagen is expressed in all life forms classified under the animal kingdom. Right from sponges, the simplest multicellular animal which expresses genes for the formation of at least two types of collagens, to the various vertebrates, in which collagen is a major component of various connective tissues, thereby accounting for roughly a quarter of the whole-body protein in humans [20]. The basic triple helical pattern has been partially carried over into the architectures of other complex molecules in higher organisms, with complex physiologies. Evolutionary branching which was partially driven by chromosomal duplication has resulted in a plethora of collagen types, which are genetically distinct. There are 29 types of collagens that have been identified so far [21]. Although the exact function of many types of collagens is yet to be confirmed, the role and presence of collagen throughout the body is unmistakable. However, it is known that collagen types I, II and III represent the majority (approx. 80–90%) of the total body collagen. They are known to provide mechanical and tensile strength to the skin and various other organs. The ability of fully developed collagen to integrate hydroxyapatites and undergo mineralization to amalgamate with solid structures such as bones and teeth, combined with its nature of elasticity and strength makes it a very desirable candidate to be used as a primary component of biomaterials with various applications [22]. Biomaterials are defined as synthetic components that may be transplanted into body tissue as a part of a medical device. Biomaterials can also be employed to replace an organ or a part of it, thereby aiding it in its physiological and mechanical functions [23].

Despite the wide range in the types of collagens, only a handful of them are actually utilized for the production of collagen-based biomaterials. Fibril forming collagens, such as type I, which also happens to be the most abundant collagen in mammals, is often employed for construction of collagen-based biomaterials for various purposes such as wound healing and tissue engineering, and even 3D bioprinting of collagen-based structures or scaffolds [24]. Collagen can be extracted from any animal's tissue including vertebrate's skin and tendons, porcine skin, gut, bladder mucosa, rat tails, as well as invertebrates' sponges and corals. The extracted collagen can show a slight difference in some characteristics, depending on the source of the animal, and the tissue. It has been found that the use of collagen from marine sources [25–28] has advantages over those obtained from terrestrial organisms, such as being environmentally sustainable, high production of collagen, non-toxicity, and ease of absorption thanks to its lower molecular weight. However, occurrence of allergies and transmission of disease can hamper the use of collagen obtained from animal sources, thereby the application of recombination technology was duly suggested, wherein yeast and *Escherichia coli* were transfected to produce recombinant collagens [29].

3.1 Collagen and biomaterials

Biomedicine is currently seeing an increase in the use and integration of collagen-based scaffold and biomaterials in its applications. The technology aids the creation of biomaterials which exhibit biomimicry of the complex native tissues and organs. Decellularized collagen and refined scaffolds are the two categories into which collagen-based biomaterials are categorized. While the decellularized collagen structures retain most of the structural and functional properties of the tissue from which it is derived from, refined scaffolds are mostly obtained from the purification and polymerization of collagen. Decellularized collagen exhibits biomimicry the best [30]. Tissue grafts for tissue engineering, self-assembled hydrogels, freeze dried sponges, collagen films and tubes are some commonly used collagen-based biomaterials.

Tissue grafts are one of the most commonly used collagen scaffolds. Due to their resemblance to the native tissues, along with the ability to promote cell attachment and spatiotemporal organization of the cells, tissue grafts have been demonstrated as the most convenient and effective implantable devices [31]. Self-assembled hydrogels are generally used in the form of cell carriers, and injectables. They are often reliable for soft tissue treatment, for they resemble the structures on polymerization to form a fibrillar hydrogel structure, which is held together by ionic and hydrophobic bonds, thus aiding the entrapment of fluids, making it conducive for the exchange of ions and metabolites in the environment created [32]. Collagen type I hydrogels in combination with the appropriate precursor cells have been extensively used for the repair and as a structural and mechanical support for the attachment and stable growth of tissues such as skin to treat burns [33], cardiac myocytes [34], neurons [35], ocular tissues [36], etc. Collagen type I and type II hydrogels have often been used in combination for the treatment and repair of osteochondral tissues, and cartilage [37, 38]. Collagen scaffolds that can be easily used as grafts for various clinical purposes are created by the freeze-drying technique, wherein, collagen on undergoing freezing in a controlled environment, is trapped within the ice crystals formed, and is porous enough to facilitate cell migration, attachment, and growth [39]. So far, a variety of cell populations have been used to improve the bioactivity of the collagen sponge, and the experiments performed have shown encouraging results both *in vivo* and *in vitro*. Collagen scaffolds, integrated with glycosaminoglycan and fibrin networks have demonstrated their ability to enhance osteogenesis, and induce osteogenic and chondrogenic differentiation [40]. It was also established that these scaffolds are also used to aid in bone regeneration [41], vascularisation [42], and skin wound healing [43]. As discussed earlier, collagen and its biomaterials have already been well established in the biomedical field for their potential bioactivities. The integration of such collagen, with nanoparticles, which in itself has found extensive applications in the field of treatment and drug delivery, has piqued the interest of the scientific community for their potential synergistic activity to enhance wound healing. The synthesis and current application of this amalgamation is discussed further.

4. Nano collagen synthesis

Nano collagen is the term used to describe collagen brought down to the nanoscale range. This substance has the desirable properties of both nanoparticles, such as a high ratio between the surface to volume of the particle, and collagen, with its wound healing properties of biomaterials, and their functions simultaneously. The downscaling of the size of the collagen fibers, is beneficial in terms of the penetration, and wound accessibility to initiate wound healing [44]. Nano collagen is produced through various chemical, physical, and self-assembly methods, such as emulsification, complex coacervation, phase separation, nano spray drying, desolvation and many other techniques. The following section explains briefly the most popular techniques employed. Nano collagen fibers are produced through the following techniques: (a) electrospinning (b) nano emulsion (c) electrospray deposition (d) milling (as shown in **Figure 2**, **Table 1**).

4.1 Electrospinning

Electrospinning is one of the methods used to create nano collagen fibers, wherein nanofibers are created from polymeric solutions in the presence of an electrostatic field. Electrospinning is achieved by charging a spinneret to high voltages and low current, and then adding droplets of the polymeric solution. As a result, the surface becomes highly charged, and elongates to form a conical shape, which is called the Taylor cone. The conical form is a result of the electrostatic repulsion between the charged droplet surface and columbic forces from the spinneret. At a specific threshold of the electric field, the electrostatic forces are strong enough to overcome the surface tension holding the Taylor cone, thus creating the fibers by stretching the cone, whipping it. This process is generally preferred to create nano fibers, because it is cost effective, and can produce nano collagen scaffolds for various purposes including tissues engineering, tissue repair and regeneration [47], and matrices that mimic the native ECM. The fibers produced through electrospinning are dry, and devoid of any solvent molecules, which are then collected in a metallic collector, which also determines the shape [51]. Over a period of time, electrospun collagen nanofibers have been endowed with certain 'smart' abilities, to improve their applications. Some smart abilities include response to external stimuli such as change in pH, exposure to light, and magnetic fields, etc., retaining a shape memory, self-cleaning, and some more [46].

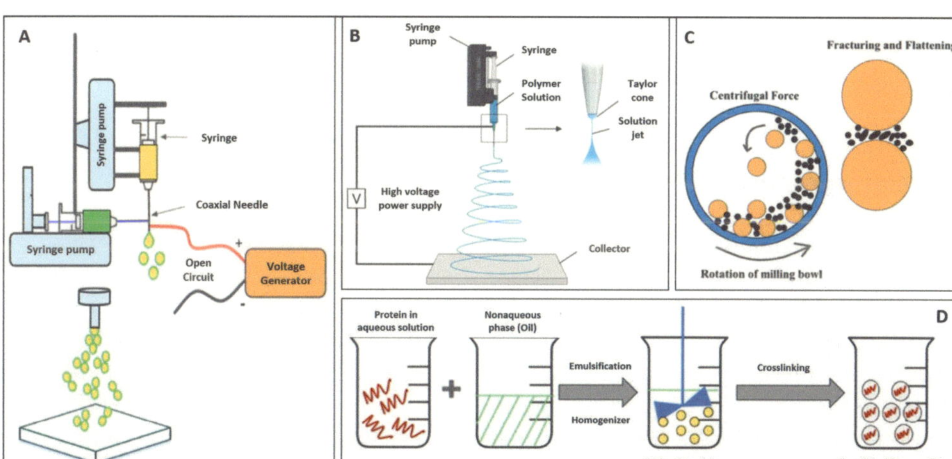

Figure 2.
(A) Electrospraying—after applying a high voltage to the protein solution, a liquid jet stream is released via a nozzle (coaxial needle), generating an aerosolized droplet. To ensure that the polymer solution comes out of the syringe as NP, a high voltage is provided to it. (B) Electrospinning—at a high voltage and low current in the spinneret, collagen polymer solution added dropwise. The Taylor cone is formed at such conditions. The columbic forces also cause the dehydration of the ejected polymer thereby resulting in thin and dry fibers of nano collagen. (C) Milling—the application of mechanical energy through the spinning of a milling bowl breaks down a polymer substance into finer NPs. Milling balls are used to conduct high-energy mechanical impacts to break down polymers utilizing centrifugal force. (D) Nanoemulsion—the emulsion is formed by the mechanical agitation of two immiscible liquid phases, one of which has the protein, and the other in which the drug is dissolved. Figures A, C, and D are reproduced with permission from [11]. Figure B is reproduced with permission from [45].

Preparation method	Principle	Advantage	Limitation	References
Electrospraying	Uses electrostatic field to create nano collagen fibers from a polymeric solution of collagen	Can be upscaled for industrial purposes; ease of particle synthesis due to single step process; formation of dry particles	Reduced flow; can degrade some macromolecules	[46]
Electrospinning	Uses a high voltage difference to generate dispersible nanoparticles from collagen solute	Can produce fine fibers of collagen; Emulates ECM closely; cost effective	Time consuming	[47]
Milling	Uses mechanical energy to break down a polymeric material of collagen to nanoparticle sizes	Economical; easy experimentation; controllable nanoparticle size	Chamber has to be cooled due to heat release; cannot control nanoparticle shape	[48]
Nanoemulsion	Uses mechanical agitation to form nanoemulsions by the combination of two immiscible liquids in different phases.	Simple process; easy recovery; high flexibility and selectivity	Requires appropriate surfactant due to unstable thermodynamic nature; the organic solvent needs to be removed, for the residues may be toxic	[49, 50]

Table 1.
Collagen nanoparticle preparation methods, their principles, advantages and limitations.

4.2 Electrospray deposition

As the name suggests, electrospray deposition is a process which involves the spraying of nano collagen solution as a fine mist onto a specific target. This method is mostly used for the applications of nanoparticles in the biomedical field for pharmaceutical application. This is mostly because, in this technique, collagen is used in its particle form. It is then sprayed through a nozzle onto a target with a high negative voltage, in the form of a fine mist. The solvent of the collagen particles generally evaporates on deposition onto the target surface, leaving an even spread of nano collagen particles, making it ideal for drug delivery purposes. This evaporation prevents the aggregation of molecules, and thus reduces the risk of contamination [52].

4.3 Milling

Milling is a process in which nano collagen is produced by the application of great amounts of mechanical stress onto a polymeric solution of collagen, to form particles of the nano scale range. This process is one of the most inexpensive methods for the large-scale production of nano collagen [53]. The mechanical energy along with the kinetic energy in the milling container also produces large amounts of heat, which can lead to the denaturation of collagen [54]. Therefore, this generation of heat is contained by performing this process at cryogenic temperatures, with the use of liquid nitrogen, thereby preserving the integrity of collagen.

4.4 Nanoemulsion

Nanoemulsion is a method used to integrate collagen with nanoparticles in a droplet form. Two immiscible liquids in different phases, i.e., oil-in-water-phase (oil is dispersed in water) and water-in-oil phase (water is dispersed in oil) when combined, form a concoction called an emulsion. Nanoemulsions differ from emulsions in their size ranges. The size of a nanoemulsion droplet ranges from 20 to 200 nm, while a normal emulsion droplet size is around 1 μm [55]. An aqueous phase with collagen, and a hydrophilic surfactant in water, is mixed with an organic phase with a lipophilic surfactant in a solvent that is immiscible in water and is continuously agitated under room temperature conditions to produce a uniform emulsion system. Nano collagen emulsion particles are then obtained by combining this emulsion system with a heated oil in a drop-by-drop manner [56]. Nanoemulsions naturally tend to penetrate deep into the tissue to deposit active compounds. This property has been exploited for purposes such as drug delivery in pharmaceutical, food and cosmetic industries. The same properties can be attributed to the collagen Nanoemulsion droplets to enhance the wound healing mechanism and speed up the process. The production of collagen nanoemulsions has increased greatly along with their application mainly in the field of cosmetics and drug delivery due to the technological advantages it offers for the manufacturers [57].

5. Applications

5.1 Bone grafting

Collagen is a major component of the bone matrix. Bone formation is facilitated by the osteoblasts, which are involved in the production of collagen type I protein. The ECM supports the collagen fibers (50–500 nm) synthesized by the osteoblasts. The hydroxyapatite crystals are then deposited on these collagen fibers, leading to the hardening and maturation of the bone [58]. This mechanism can be exploited for the purposes of bone remodeling, in the case of a grave bone injury such as a compound fracture. A collagen scaffold can be grafted onto the damaged tissue area, to provide a solid support onto which the apatite crystals can be deposited, to increase the speed and efficiency of new bone formation. It is thus prudent that the collagen scaffold mimics native collagen fibers to achieve successful bone grafting and promote optimal bone regrowth.

It is well known that bone related tissue trauma is difficult to treat and is a time-consuming process, due to the complexity of the bone healing process itself, and the loss of bone from non-sterile wounds, creating a high risk and susceptibility for infections. Cardoso et al., proposed the use of silver nanoparticles stabilized with type I collagen to form nano collagen biomaterials (AgNPcol) for the collagen scaffold to support rapid bone remodeling. This was an optimal solution for the problem of infections caused due to the non-sterility of the bone wounds. The silver nanoparticles in the collagen also showed anti-microbial activity against a number of microorganisms. Thereby proving to be effective in wound healing. The developed cells also showed no signs of cell toxicity [59]. In another study by Sun et al., collagen scaffolds were infused with AgNPs along with BMP2, a bone morphogenic protein to improve the bone healing process effectively. The role of silver nanoparticles in antibacterial property was already established. However, the incorporation of the bone morphogenic protein induced an increase in the expression of runt related transcription factor 2, osteopontin and osteonectin, which are known to accelerate the differentiation of the bone marrow derived mesenchymal stromal cells, thereby proving the therapeutic potential of nano collagen in bone grafting, and healing [60].

Poor development of alveolar ridge after tooth extraction is an issue faced by most dental patients due to the lack of oral hygiene or knowledge about it. Wang et al., in their research, proposed the usage of artificial nano collagen bone implants. This was done to support the alveolar ridge post extraction of tooth. The implantation was followed by a CT scan to track the bone mineral density progressively. It was found that the implanted nano collagen bone has successfully fused with the native alveolar bridge. It also showed an increase in the overall bone mineral density [61].

5.2 Nerve tissue

Treatment of damaged nerve tissues has been a topic of interest for many researchers. This can be attributed to the inability of terminally differentiated neurons to undergo further cell division and also the fact that the nervous system controls and coordinates most of our body's processes. Damage or injury caused to the nerve tissue can seriously impair many functions of the body. Autografts of the nerve tissue has been performed in some cases. However, this has proven to be more challenging, due to the shortage of the donor sites, or occurrence of deformities. This has fuelled the search for alternative methods or materials to treat nerve damages effectively. The extensive study on collagen and nano collagen has tested the ability of collagen to act as an effective scaffold and promote cell attachment and growth [62]. Collagen has been used in the manufacture of nerve guidance conduits to aid the nerve regeneration in small nerve gaps of 2–3 cm across the peripheral nerve tissue. The use of collagen hydrogels for the treatment of lesions in the central nervous system effectively has been demonstrated by Orive et al. [63]. Further degradation of the nerve tissues can be prevented on injection of collagen nanospheres, which have the potential to deliver therapeutic drugs, and other stem cells for structural support as well [64]. Zhang et al., illustrated the application of collagen—nano size β tricalcium phosphate, together with growth factors of nerves and some collagen fibers, for the treatment of facial nerve repair and regeneration. Improved action potential was seen in the muscles, along with the formation of thicker myelin sheath, making it a highly promising avenue for further innovation and studies in nerve regeneration [65].

5.3 Articular cartilage

Articular cartilage covers the edge of a bone, and it is a connective tissue which forms a synovial joint that provides low frictional surface and enables the smooth movement of the joint. So, any damage to the articular cartilage results in acute pain during the movement of the joint. However, unlike most tissues in the body, articular cartilage lacks the potential to heal itself by replacing damaged areas in the tissue with new cells. This is mainly due to its avascular nature, i.e., there is no direct blood supply to the cartilage, thereby making it a difficult to heal by targeting therapeutic drugs. Treatment for articular cartilage necessitates surgical intervention techniques such as chondrocytes implantation and osteochondral transplant. However, the high cost and numerous other risk factors of patients has given rise to much needed research in the field of cartilage tissue engineering [66].

Cartilage tissue engineering employs the use of 3D bioprinting for the creation of collagen 3D scaffolds, which are then treated *in vitro* to make them suitable for implantation. The application of 3D bioprinting techniques along with the nano collagen scaffolds effectively reduces the requirement of a cartilage transplantation from a donor, along with the need for other less effective surgical options. A collagen-hydroxyapatite hydrogel nanocomposite was developed and effectively used in an investigation which showed promising results. Hydrogel composite was found to be suitable to facilitate fluid transport, and also thermally stable up to a temperature of 90°C [67]. Jiang et al., illustrated a different approach to stimulate the differentiation of the chondrocytes in the articular cartilage in order to initiate the repair mechanisms. The inhibition of chondrocyte dedifferentiation was achieved by the use of nano hydroxyapatite collagen scaffolds [68].

5.4 Skin wound healing

The process of wound healing involves four steps viz., hemostasis, inflammation, proliferation, and remodeling which occur in a sequential order [69]. Disruption of any of these steps will make the process lengthy. The main issue involved in wound healing is infection by pathogens that results in inflammation, interrupting the healing process [45]. Schimek et al., developed full-thickness skin equivalents (ftSEs) to hold the 96-well cell culture [70]. Collagen powder can be used as the dermal substitute as they are part of the ECM that shows slow biodegradation and accelerates wound healing [45]. Collagen with nanoparticles is widely used in therapy. Munish et al., used collagen granules for the diabetic foot ulcer treatment and the results were compared with the saline dressing. The study demonstrated that the wound, when treated with collagen showed a speedy recovery [71]. In another study, Akturk et al., developed gold nanoparticles (AuNPs) based collagen scaffold, and they were incorporated into the cross- linked collagen scaffolds. It was found that it helps in enhancing the stability against enzymatic degradation and increases the tensile strength [72]. The main advantage includes the absence of rejection and the fact that they can reduce the inflammation in and around the wound. Apart from gold nanoparticles, the use of silver as an antimicrobial agent has also been of great interest recently. Silver nanoparticles (AgNPs) are usually used in the treatment of burns and infection as they are known to demonstrate antibacterial property. There is sufficient evidence to prove that the bacterial resistance against AgNPs may not be a matter of concern, for AgNPs are known to hinder quorum sensing mechanisms in bacteria [45].

Collagen-based dermal scaffolds are coated with silver nanoparticles that act as antimicrobial dressing without having any toxic side effects. Nano silver reacts with gram-negative and gram-positive bacteria, causing damage to the intracellular structure. The positively charged silver nanoparticles react with negatively charged bacterial surfaces leading to the disruption of the inner membrane. During electrospinning, the synthesized silver nano particles are incorporated into the collagen nano fibers. The *in vitro* results prove that the AuNPs and AgNPs can provide the antimicrobial conditions for wound healing. The rate of wound healing in case of collagen composite nanofiber mat was significantly higher compared to the regular nanofiber collagen [44].

5.5 Drug delivery

Collagen nanoparticles have shown promise as treatment carriers [73]. The recent trends in nanotechnology research and development aims to create collagen scaffolds that deliver the drug to the specific site and are released in a controlled manner [74]. Gold nanoparticles with different concentrations of gold (Au) was synthesized and coated onto collagen to form an amalgamation of nanoparticles and collagen (Au-Hp-Col). This amalgamation was found to be effective in the delivery of the drug Doxorubicin [70]. Poloxamer 407 (PM) is a polymer soluble in water used in the delivery of ophthalmic drugs like Ketorolac Tromethamine (KT). The PM is incorporated into the cellulose nano collagen particles that showed controlled release of the drug *in vitro* [73]. One of the case studies demonstrated the use of collagen nanoparticles in drug delivery to treat tumors. Collagen is a major component of the tumor microenvironment. The study involved the development of tumor spheroids based on collagen that are optimized using cell lines like 95-D, U87, HCT116 [75]. It was observed that the conjugated nanoparticles showed greater penetration into the gel matrix and were able to gain access to the tumor cells [76].

5.6 Vascular grafting

Cardiovascular disease is the major cause of death worldwide [77]. These disorders are caused by reduced blood flow by blockage of blood vessels [78, 79]. Presently, the saphenous vein, the internal thoracic artery, and autologous vessels are used as grafts which are known to perform better than the synthetic alternative [80]. However, their limited availability and invasive harvest make them unsuitable for use. Tissue-engineered vascular grafts (TEVG) are currently used in order to overcome these limitations [48]. TEVG makes use of modern technology for the construction of vascular medical implants. The collagen along with the other components are used as a scaffold in the preparation of the TEVGs. In a previous study, Park et al., described a poly-epsilon-caprolactone (PCL) vascular graft, and its suitability for healing process. It was observed that the graft undergoes gradual degradation replaced by natural blood vessels. Collagen is also incorporated on to the inner layer and silica (sol-gel-derived ceramic) into the outer layer of PCL to improve the vascular response [49].

6. Conclusion

This chapter conclusively describes the importance and role of nanoparticles-based collagen biomaterials in the treatment of various wounds. The ECM is mainly comprised of collagen, which provides support and elasticity against mechanical stress. While collagen in itself is useful in the form of various biomaterials like scaffold s and hydrogels, the introduction of nanotechnology to it comes with its own set of challenges as well as advantages. The reduction of collagen to the nano particle's sizes, giving it a large surface-to-volume ratio, is known to increase its efficiency of dealing with mechanical stress, thereby making it a viable option for treatment of wounds. Multiple research studies are conducted on wound healing using various materials and methods to reduce risk infection and aid in speedy recovery of the patient. The antimicrobial properties of nanoparticles of various elements such as gold and silver has already been proven, which can be further exploited in the effective treatment of wounds and injuries, in combination with collagen. The current challenge lies in the effective incorporation of nanoparticles and collagen in the production of nano collagen biomaterials, upscaling the production of nano collagen and making it affordable to the general public.

Acknowledgements

NM thank Global Innovation and Technology Alliance (GITA), Department of Science and Technology (DST), India [Project Number-GITA/DST/TWN/P-95/2021], and Indian Council of Medical Research (ICMR), (Project Number-ITR/Ad-hoc/43/2020-21, ID No. 2020-3286) Government of India, India for financial support.

Conflict of interest

The authors declare no conflict of interest.

Author details

Kausalya Neelavara Makkithaya[1†], Sharmila Nadumane[1†], Guan-Yu Zhuo[2], Sanjiban Chakrabarty[3*] and Nirmal Mazumder[1*]

1 Department of Biophysics, Manipal School of Life Sciences, Manipal Academy of Higher Education, Manipal, Karnataka, India

2 Institute of New Drug Development, China Medical University, Taichung, Taiwan

3 Department of Cell and Molecular Biology, Manipal School of Life Sciences, Manipal Academy of Higher Education, Manipal, Karnataka, India

*Address all correspondence to: sanjiban.c@manipal.edu and nirmaluva@gmail.com

† Equal contribution.

References

[1] Albaugh VL, Mukherjee K, Barbul A. Proline precursors and collagen synthesis: Biochemical challenges of nutrient supplementation and wound healing. The Journal of Nutrition. 2017;**147**(11):2011-2017. DOI: 10.3945/jn.117.256404

[2] Witte MB, Barbul A. General principles of wound healing. Surgical Clinics of North America. 1997;**77**(3):509-528. DOI: 10.1016/S0039-6109(05)70566-1

[3] Felician FF, Yu RH, Li MZ, Li CJ, Chen HQ, Jiang Y, et al. The wound healing potential of collagen peptides derived from the jellyfish Rhopilema esculentum. Chinese Journal of Traumatology. 2019;**22**(1):12-20. DOI: 10.1016/j.cjtee.2018.10.004

[4] Lin H, Zheng Z, Yuan J, Zhang C, Cao W, Qin X. Collagen peptides derived from Sipunculus nudus accelerate wound healing. Molecules. 2021;**26**(5):1385. DOI: 10.3390/molecules26051385

[5] Lim YS, Ok YJ, Hwang SY, Kwak JY, Yoon S. Marine collagen as a promising biomaterial for biomedical applications. Marine Drugs. 2019;**17**(8):467. DOI: 10.3390/md17080467

[6] Wang Y, Tan H, Hui X. Biomaterial scaffolds in regenerative therapy of the central nervous system. BioMed Research International. 2018;**1**:1-19. DOI: 10.1155/2018/7848901

[7] Kolahalam LA, Viswanath IK, Diwakar BS, Govindh B, Reddy V, Murthy YL. Review on nanomaterials: Synthesis and applications. Materials Today: Proceedings. 2019;**18**:2182-2190. DOI: 10.1016/j.matpr.2019.07.371

[8] Ngiam M, Nguyen LT, Liao S, Chan CK, Ramakrishna S. Biomimetic nanostructured materials potential regulators for osteogenesis. Annals of the Academy of Medicine, Singapore. 2011;**40**(5):213-212

[9] Freitas RA Jr. What is nanomedicine? Nanomedicine: Nanotechnology, Biology and Medicine. 2005;**1**(1):2-9. DOI: 10.1016/j.nano.2004.11.003

[10] Bhushan B, Baumann. . In: Bhushan B, editor. Springer Handbook of Nanotechnology. Berlin: Springer; 2007

[11] Mihai MM, Dima MB, Dima B, Holban AM. Nanomaterials for wound healing and infection control. Materials. 2019;**12**(13):2176. DOI: 10.3390/ma12132176

[12] Chakrabarti S, Chattopadhyay P, Islam J, Ray S, Raju PS, Mazumder B. Aspects of nanomaterials in wound healing. Current Drug Delivery. 2019;**16**(1):26-41. DOI: 10.2174/1567201815666180918110134

[13] Lu XY, Wu DC, Li ZJ, Chen GQ. Polymer nanoparticles. Progress in Molecular Biology and Translational Science. 2011;**104**:299-323. DOI: 10.1016/B978-0-12-416020-0.00007-3

[14] Gupta A. Nanoemulsions. In: Nanoparticles for Biomedical Applications. Amsterdam: Elsevier; 2020. pp. 371-384. DOI: 10.1016/B978-0-12-816662-8.00021-7

[15] Patel MR, Patel RB, Thakore SD. Nanoemulsion in drug delivery. In: Applications of Nanocomposite Materials in Drug Delivery. Cambridge: Woodhead Publishing; 2018. pp. 667-700. DOI: 10.1016/B978-0-12-813741-3.00030-3

[16] Rajendran NK, Kumar SS, Houreld NN, Abrahamse H. A review on nanoparticle based treatment for wound healing. Journal of Drug Delivery Science and Technology. 2018;**44**:421-430. DOI: 10.1016/j.jddst.2018.01.009

[17] Zhao DH, Yang J, Yao MH, Li CQ, Zhang B, Zhu D, et al. An in situ synthesis of silver nanoparticle-loaded genetically engineered polypeptide nanogels for antibacterial and wound healing applications. Dalton Transactions. 2020;**49**(34):12049-12055. DOI: 10.1039/D0DT00751J

[18] Parenteau N. Skin: The first tissue-engineered products. Scientific American. 1999;**280**(4):83-85

[19] Persikov AV, Ramshaw JA, Kirkpatrick A, Brodsky B. Electrostatic interactions involving lysine make major contributions to collagen triple-helix stability. Biochemistry. 2005;**44**(5):1414-1422. DOI: 10.1021/bi048216r

[20] Viguet-Carrin S, Garnero P, Delmas PD. The role of collagen in bone strength. Osteoporosis International. 2006;**17**(3):319-336. DOI: 10.1007/s00198-005-2035-9

[21] Mk G, Ra H. Collagens. Cell and Tissue Research. 2010;**339**:247-257

[22] Sionkowska A, Skrzyński S, Śmiechowski K, Kołodziejczak A. The review of versatile application of collagen. Polymers for Advanced Technologies. 2017;**28**(1):4-9. DOI: 10.1002/pat.3842

[23] Zhang X, Williams D, editors. Definitions of Biomaterials for the Twenty-First Century. Amsterdam: Elsevier; 2019

[24] Chattopadhyay S, Raines RT. Collagen-based biomaterials for wound healing. Biopolymers. 2014;**101**(8):821-833. DOI: 10.1002/bip.22486

[25] Ehrlich H, Deutzmann R, Brunner E, Cappellini E, Koon H, Solazzo C, et al. Mineralization of the metre-long biosilica structures of glass sponges is templated on hydroxylated collagen. Nature Chemistry. 2010;**2**(12):1084-1088. DOI: 10.1038/nchem.899

[26] Orgel JP, Sella I, Madhurapantula RS, Antipova O, Mandelberg Y, Kashman Y, et al. Molecular and ultrastructural studies of a fibrillar collagen from octocoral (Cnidaria). Journal of Experimental Biology. 2017;**220**(18):3327-3335. DOI: 10.1242/jeb.163824

[27] Tziveleka LA, Ioannou E, Tsiourvas D, Berillis P, Foufa E, Roussis V. Collagen from the marine sponges Axinella cannabina and Suberites carnosus: Isolation and morphological, biochemical, and biophysical characterization. Marine Drugs. 2017;**15**(6):152. DOI: 10.3390/md15060152

[28] Rahman MA. An overview of the medical applications of marine skeletal matrix proteins. Marine Drugs. 2016;**14**(9):167. DOI: 10.3390/md14090167

[29] Olsen D, Yang C, Bodo M, Chang R, Leigh S, Baez J, et al. Recombinant collagen and gelatin for drug delivery. Advanced Drug Delivery Reviews. 2003;**55**(12):1547-1567. DOI: 10.1016/j.addr.2003.08.008

[30] Zitnay JL, Reese SP, Tran G, Farhang N, Bowles RD, Weiss JA. Fabrication of dense anisotropic collagen scaffolds using biaxial compression. Acta Biomaterialia. 2018;**65**:76-87. DOI: 10.1016/j.actbio.2017.11.017

[31] Song JJ, Ott HC. Organ engineering based on decellularized matrix scaffolds. Trends in Molecular Medicine. 2011;**17**(8):424-432. DOI: 10.1016/j.molmed.2011.03.005

[32] Abou Neel EA, Cheema U, Knowles JC, Brown RA, Nazhat SN. Use of multiple unconfined compression for control of collagen gel scaffold density and mechanical properties. Soft Matter. 2006;**2**(11):986-992. DOI: 10.1039/B609784G

[33] Pensalfini M, Ehret AE, Stüdeli S, Marino D, Kaech A, Reichmann E, et al. Factors affecting the mechanical behavior of collagen hydrogels for skin tissue engineering. Journal of the Mechanical Behavior of Biomedical Materials. 2017;**69**:85-97. DOI: 10.1016/j.jmbbm.2016.12.004

[34] Tulloch NL, Muskheli V, Razumova MV, Korte FS, Regnier M, Hauch KD, et al. Growth of engineered human myocardium with mechanical loading and vascular coculture. Circulation Research. 2011;**109**(1):47-59. DOI: 10.1161/CIRCRESAHA.110.237206

[35] Koppes AN, Keating KW, McGregor AL, Koppes RA, Kearns KR, Ziemba AM, et al. Robust neurite extension following exogenous electrical stimulation within single walled carbon nanotube-composite hydrogels. Acta Biomaterialia. 2016;**39**:34-43. DOI: 10.1016/j.actbio.2016.05.014

[36] Mi S, Chen B, Wright B, Connon CJ. Plastic compression of a collagen gel forms a much improved scaffold for ocular surface tissue engineering over conventional collagen gels. Journal of Biomedical Materials Research Part A. 2010;**95**(2):447-453. DOI: 10.1002/jbm.a.32861

[37] Lu Z, Doulabi BZ, Huang C, Bank RA, Helder MN. Collagen type II enhances chondrogenesis in adipose tissue–derived stem cells by affecting cell shape. Tissue Engineering Part A. 2010;**16**(1):81-90. DOI: 10.1089/ten.tea.2009.0222

[38] Hu D, Shan X. Effects of different concentrations of type-I collagen hydrogel on the growth and differentiation of chondrocytes. Experimental and Therapeutic Medicine. 2017;**14**(6):5411-5416. DOI: 10.3892/etm.2017.5202

[39] Haugh MG, Murphy CM, O'Brien FJ. Novel freeze-drying methods to produce a range of collagen–glycosaminoglycan scaffolds with tailored mean pore sizes. Tissue Engineering Part C: Methods. 2010;**16**(5):887-894. DOI: 10.1089/ten.tec.2009.0422

[40] Keogh MB, Partap S, Daly JS, O'Brien FJ. Three hours of perfusion culture prior to 28 days of static culture, enhances osteogenesis by human cells in a collagen GAG scaffold. Biotechnology and Bioengineering. 2011;**108**(5):1203-1210. DOI: 10.1002/bit.23032

[41] Quinlan E, Thompson EM, Matsiko A, O'Brien FJ, López-Noriega A. Long-term controlled delivery of rhBMP-2 from collagen–hydroxyapatite scaffolds for superior bone tissue regeneration. Journal of Controlled Release. 2015;**207**:112-119. DOI: 10.1016/j.jconrel.2015.03.028

[42] Markowicz M, Koellensperger E, Neuss S, Koenigschulte S, Bindler C, Pallua N. Human bone marrow mesenchymal stem cells seeded on modified collagen improved dermal regeneration *in vivo*. Cell Transplantation. 2006;**15**(8-9):723-732. DOI: 10.3727/000000006783464408

[43] Onuma-Ukegawa M, Bhatt K, Hirai T, Kaburagi H, Sotome S, Wakabayashi Y, et al. Bone marrow stromal cells combined

with a honeycomb collagen sponge facilitate neurite elongation *in vitro* and neural restoration in the hemisected rat spinal cord. Cell Transplantation. 2015;7:1283-1297. DOI: 10.3727/096368914X682134

[44] Naskar A, Kim KS. Recent advances in nanomaterial-based wound-healing therapeutics. Pharmaceutics. 2020;**12**(6):499. DOI: 10.3727/096368914X682134

[45] Lo S, Fauzi MB. Current update of collagen nanomaterials—Fabrication, characterisation and its applications: A review. Pharmaceutics. 2021;**13**(3):316. DOI: 10.3390/pharmaceutics13030316

[46] Xue J, Wu T, Dai Y, Xia Y. Electrospinning and electrospun nanofibers: Methods, materials, and applications. Chemical Reviews. 2019;**119**(8):5298-5415. DOI: 10.1021/acs.chemrev.8b00593

[47] Law JX, Liau LL, Saim A, Yang Y, Idrus R. Electrospun collagen nanofibers and their applications in skin tissue engineering. Tissue Engineering and Regenerative Medicine. 2017;**14**(6):699-718. DOI: 10.1007/s13770-017-0075-9

[48] Park S, Kim J, Lee MK, Park C, Jung HD, Kim HE, et al. Fabrication of strong, bioactive vascular grafts with PCL/collagen and PCL/silica bilayers for small-diameter vascular applications. Materials & Design. 2019;**181**:108079. DOI: 10.1016/j.matdes.2019.108079

[49] Morgan PW. Interfacial polymerisation. In: Encyclopedia of Polymer science and Technology. New Jersey: John Wiley & Sons, Ltd; 2011

[50] Wang G, Uludag H. Recent developments in nanoparticle-based drug delivery and targeting systems with emphasis on protein-based nanoparticles. Expert Opinion on Drug Delivery. 2008;**5**(5):499-515. DOI: 10.1517/17425247.5.5.499

[51] Sundaramurthi D, Krishnan UM, Sethuraman S. Electrospun nanofibers as scaffolds for skin tissue engineering. Polymer Reviews. 2014;**54**(2):348-376. DOI: 10.1080/15583724.2014.881374

[52] Nagarajan U, Kawakami K, Zhang S, Chandrasekaran B, Nair BU. Fabrication of solid collagen nanoparticles using electrospray deposition. Chemical and Pharmaceutical Bulletin. 2014;**62**(5):422-428. DOI: 10.1248/cpb.c13-01004

[53] Mhetar SK, Ashok Nerle A, Patil RL, Pawar RA, Patil MM, Shinde HT. Cost effective ball milling machine for producing nanopowder. International Journal of Research in Engineering and Technology. 2017;**4**:330-334

[54] Kumar M, Xiong X, Wan Z, Sun Y, Tsang DC, Gupta J, et al. Ball milling as a mechanochemical technology for fabrication of novel biochar nanomaterials. Bioresource Technology. 2020;**2**:123613. DOI: 10.1016/j.biortech.2020.123613

[55] Yukuyama MN, Ghisleni DD, Pinto TD, Bou-Chacra NA. Nanoemulsion: Process selection and application in cosmetics—A review. International Journal of Cosmetic Science. 2016;**38**(1):13-24. DOI: 10.1111/ics.12260

[56] Singh AN, Yethiraj A. Liquid–liquid phase separation as the second step of complex coacervation. The Journal of Physical Chemistry B. 2021;**125**(12):3023-3031. DOI: 10.1021/acs.jpcb.0c07349

[57] Musazzi UM, Franzè S, Minghetti P, Casiraghi A. Emulsion versus nanoemulsion: How much is the formulative shift critical for a

cosmetic product? Drug Delivery and Translational Research. 2018;**8**(2):414-421. DOI: 10.1007/s13346-017-0390-7

[58] Katsimbri P. The biology of normal bone remodelling. European Journal of Cancer Care. 2017;**6**:e12740. DOI: 10.1111/ecc.12740

[59] Cardoso VS, Quelemes PV, Amorin A, Primo FL, Gobo GG, Tedesco AC, et al. Collagen-based silver nanoparticles for biological applications: Synthesis and characterization. Journal of Nanobiotechnology. 2014;**1**:1-9. DOI: 10.1111/ecc.12740

[60] Sun CY, Che YJ, Lu SJ. Preparation and application of collagen scaffold-encapsulated silver nanoparticles and bone morphogenetic protein 2 for enhancing the repair of infected bone. Biotechnology Letters. 2015;**2**:467-473. DOI: 10.1007/s10529-014-1698-8

[61] Wang CY, Zhao Y, Yang M, Wang SF. Nano-collagen artificial bone for alveolar ridge preservation in the Kazakh from Xinjiang Tacheng region. Chinese Journal of Tissue Engineering Research. 2015;**12**:1864. DOI: 10.3969/j.issn.2095-4344.2015.12.012

[62] Mohamadi F, Ebrahimi-Barough S, Reza Nourani M, Ali Derakhshan M, Goodarzi V, Sadegh Nazockdast M, et al. Electrospun nerve guide scaffold of poly (ε-caprolactone)/collagen/nanobioglass: An *in vitro* study in peripheral nerve tissue engineering. Journal of Biomedical Materials Research Part A. 2017;**105**(7):1960-1972. DOI: 10.1002/jbm.a.36068

[63] Orive G, Anitua E, Pedraz JL, Emerich DF. Biomaterials for promoting brain protection, repair and regeneration. Nature Reviews Neuroscience. 2009;**10**(9):682-692. DOI: 10.1038/nrn2685

[64] Ucar B, Humpel C. Collagen for brain repair: Therapeutic perspectives. Neural regeneration research. 2018;**4**:595. DOI: 10.4103/1673-5374.230273

[65] Zhang Z, Li X, Li Z, Bai Y, Liao G, Pan J, et al. Collagen/nano-sized β-tricalcium phosphate conduits combined with collagen filaments and nerve growth factor promote facial nerve regeneration in miniature swine: An *in vivo* study. Oral Surgery, Oral Medicine, Oral Pathology and Oral Radiology. 2019;**8**(5):472-478. DOI: 10.1016/j.oooo.2018.12.006

[66] Armiento AR, Stoddart MJ, Alini M, Eglin D. Biomaterials for articular cartilage tissue engineering: Learning from biology. Acta Biomaterialia. 2018;**65**:1-20. DOI: 10.1016/j.actbio.2017.11.021

[67] Kaviani A, Zebarjad SM, Javadpour S, Ayatollahi M, Bazargan-Lari R. Fabrication and characterization of low-cost freeze-gelated chitosan/collagen/hydroxyapatite hydrogel nanocomposite scaffold. International Journal of Polymer Analysis and Characterization. 2019;**24**(3):191-203. DOI: 10.1080/1023666X.2018.1562477

[68] Jiang X, Zhong Y, Zheng L, Zhao J. Nano-hydroxyapatite/collagen film as a favorable substrate to maintain the phenotype and promote the growth of chondrocytes cultured *in vitro* Corrigendum in/10.3892/ijmm.2020.4743. International Journal of Molecular Medicine. 2018;**41**(4):2150-2158. DOI: 10.3892/ijmm.2016.2722

[69] Wallace HA, Basehore BM, Zito PM. Wound Healing Phases. In: StatPearls. Treasure Island: StatPearls Publishing; 2021

[70] Schimek K, Hsu HH, Boehme M, Kornet JJ, Marx U, Lauster R, et al. Bioengineering of a full-thickness skin equivalent in a 96-well insert format for

substance permeation studies and organ-on-a-chip applications. Bioengineering. 2018;**5**(2):43. DOI: 10.3390/bioengineering5020043

[71] Munish T, Ramneesh G, Sanjeev S, Jasdeep S, Jaspal S, Nikhil G. Comparative study of collagen based dressing and standard dressing in diabetic foot ulcer. Journal of Evolution of Medical and Dental Sciences. 2015;**4**(21):3614-3622

[72] Akturk O, Kismet K, Yasti AC, Kuru S, Duymus ME, Kaya F, et al. Collagen/gold nanoparticle nanocomposites: A potential skin wound healing biomaterial. Journal of biomaterials applications. 2016;**31**(2):283-301. DOI: 10.1177/0885328216644536

[73] You C, Li Q, Wang X, Wu P, Ho JK, Jin R, et al. Silver nanoparticle loaded collagen/chitosan scaffolds promote wound healing via regulating fibroblast migration and macrophage activation. Scientific Reports. 2017;**7**(1):1-1. DOI: 10.1038/s41598-017-10481-0

[74] Jahangirian H, Lemraski EG, Webster TJ, Rafiee-Moghaddam R, Abdollahi Y. A review of drug delivery systems based on nanotechnology and green chemistry: Green nanomedicine. International Journal of Nanomedicine. 2017;**12**:2957. DOI: 10.2147/IJN.S127683

[75] Le VM, Lang MD, Shi WB, Liu JW. A collagen-based multicellular tumor spheroid model for evaluation of the efficiency of nanoparticle drug delivery. Artificial Cells, Nanomedicine, and Biotechnology. 2016;**44**(2):540-544. DOI: 10.3109/21691401.2014.968820

[76] Zoghbi WA, Duncan T, Antman E, Barbosa M, Champagne B, Chen D, et al. Sustainable development goals and the future of cardiovascular health: A statement from the global cardiovascular disease taskforce. Journal of the American Heart Association. 2014;**3**(5):e000504. DOI: 10.1161/JAHA.114.000504

[77] Mathers CD, Loncar D. Projections of global mortality and burden of disease from 2002 to 2030. PLoS Medicine. 2006;**3**(11):e442. DOI: 10.1371/journal.pmed.0030442

[78] Arun A, Malrautu P, Laha A, Luo H, Ramakrishna S. Collagen nanoparticles in drug delivery systems and tissue engineering. Applied Sciences. 2021;**11**(23):11369. DOI: 10.3390/app112311369

[79] Mondal S, Hoang G, Manivasagan P, Moorthy MS, Phan TT, Kim HH, et al. Rapid microwave-assisted synthesis of gold loaded hydroxyapatite collagen nano-bio materials for drug delivery and tissue engineering application. Ceramics International. 2019;**45**(3):2977-2988. DOI: 10.1016/j.ceramint.2018.10.016

[80] Pashneh-Tala S, MacNeil S, Claeyssens F. The tissue-engineered vascular graft—Past, present, and future. Tissue Engineering Part B: Reviews. 2016;**22**(1):68-100. DOI: 10.1089/ten.teb.2015.0100

Chapter 4

Thermal Manipulation of Human Bone Collagen Membrane (SoftBone) and Platelet-Rich Fibrin (PRF) Membranes

Lajos Csönge, Ágnes Bozsik, Zoltán T. Bagi, Róbert Gyuris, Dóra K. Csönge and János Kónya

Abstract

Resorbable barrier membranes, including platelet-rich fibrin (PRF) and collagen membranes, can play a key role in guided bone regeneration surgeries (GBR) in dentistry. A new collagen membrane made of partially decalcified allogeneic cortical bone, termed SoftBone membrane (SB), was produced by West Hungarian Regional Tissue Bank. It can be easily adapted to diverse surfaces. Fresh and freeze-dried folded-PRF membranes were compared with freeze-dried SB. Important properties of membranes were reported (moisture content, rehydration capacity, and resistance against proteolytic enzyme). The SB exhibited the best resistance against enzymatic digestion on day 21, its weight was 34% of the original. Fresh F-PRF (folded PRF) disintegrated on the 11th day, while the freeze-dried F-PRF membrane dissolved completely on day 8. The thermal manipulation of the F-PRF membrane using freeze-drying has advantages and also disadvantages in comparison to the fresh one.

Keywords: regenerative dentistry, guided bone regeneration, F-PRF, collagen membrane, freeze-drying

1. Introduction

Collagen membranes have been utilized for decades in numerous surgical fields, including neurosurgery, abdominal surgery, othorhinolaryngology, and dental surgery [1–5].

GBR is a popular surgical process for bone augmentation before dental implantation. There were different collagen membranes historically but in recent times resorbable membranes have been mostly applied. During the resorption period, these barrier membranes can protect the submembranous bone particles from the unintended ingrowth of fibroblasts and epithelial cells (see **Figure 1**).

Therefore bone morphogenesis can remain intact, but it can be impacted by several other factors, such as local pressure and infection. Bovine xenogeneic membranes and

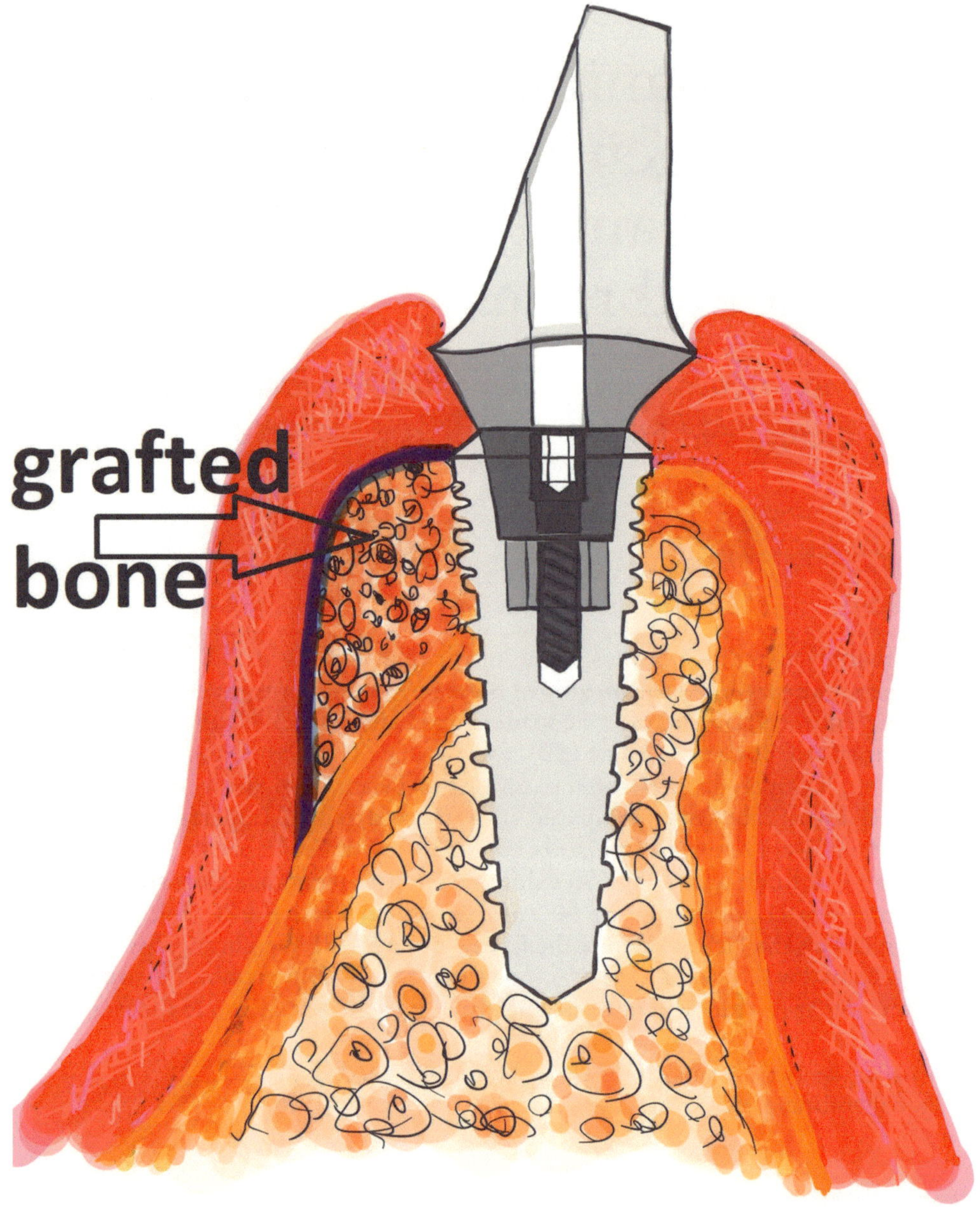

Figure 1.
Clinical application of barrier membrane (blue) in GBR. The membrane can protect the grafted bone particles from the unintended ingrowth of gingival fibroblasts and epithelial cells.

allogeneic membranes can also be found on the market. Their main advantage is the strong biomechanical properties and the ability for resorption [5–7].

The main preservation method of the collagen membranes is freeze-drying (lyophilization). The aim of this process is to decrease the water content of the tissue by under 5% so that these freeze-dried products can be stored at room temperature. Without water the autolytic enzymes cannot work, so membranes remain intact. Before or during surgery the membrane is rehydrated.

During the last two decades, the number of reports on the clinical application of different platelet-rich products in oral surgery and implant dentistry has increased. Especially those examining local tissue regeneration and include GBR either alone or in combination with particulated bone grafts. Several techniques for platelet concentrates have been introduced in the surgical field for the acceleration of tissue regeneration. Two main groups of platelet-rich products can be distinguished—(1) first-generation platelet-rich plasma (PRP) products with anticoagulants and (2) second-generation PRF products without anticoagulants. PRF can also be used as a barrier membrane in GBR similar to a collagen membrane [8–11].

The main effect of platelet-rich products is based on the theory of regenerative properties of the autologous cells, such as leukocytes (LCs), platelets (PLs), and stem cells. They release cytokines and growth factors (e.g., PDGF-platelet derived growth factor, EGF-epithelial growth factor, VEGF, and TGF-transforming growth factor) for 2–3 weeks *in vitro* playing a crucial role in bone and soft tissue regeneration. A total of 10^6/μl platelets are likely and are in the therapeutically effective range; it is 4–5 times higher than baseline platelet count values in whole blood [12].

PRF is a special mixture of individual cells entrapped in a freshly nascent fibrin clot that later serves as autoscaffold. Depending on the leukocyte or fibrin content, platelet concentrates can be classified into different categories—leukocyte and platelet-rich plasma (L-PRP); pure platelet-rich fibrin (P-PRF); leukocyte and platelet-rich fibrin (L-PRF); F-PRF; injectable i-PRF; advanced A-PRF; autologous albumin gel and platelet-rich fibrin (Alb-PRF); etc. [13–22]. Unfortunately, the names of different membranes are sometimes confusing.

The F-PRF membrane was created and published by our group [20]. It has many attractive properties (e.g., homogenous cell distribution and better biomechanical properties) in comparison to conventional methods.

Many articles describe these different PRF membranes. Their properties that have been reported include platelet number, cell number and their distribution in membranes, biomechanical properties, and cytokine distribution and their release over time. This report is not going to recapitulate these findings. Generally, PRF membranes are prepared at the bedside for immediate autologous clinical application and short-term use (for up to 14-days) but this approach somewhat limits their therapeutic value [16–23].

PRF membranes accelerate bone substitute healing and allow for earlier implant placement compared to collagen membranes, but collagen membranes can stimulate bone regeneration significantly during later stages, as was reported in a model using sheep [24].

Metabolic activity and proliferation of human osteoblast cells *in vitro* were supported to a significantly higher extent by eluates from fresh PRF membranes. Collagen and PRF membranes are suitable as scaffolds for the cultivation of human osteoblast cells *in vitro*; proliferation was significantly higher on PRF membranes and PRF clots than on BioGide® collagen membranes [25].

The PRF membrane can be applied as a sole barrier membrane only when re-entry (a second surgical flap) is not clinically required. In extensive GBR cases, PRF membranes are combined with either a collagen barrier membrane or titanium mesh. As a rule of thumb, it is always advantageous to utilize PRF on the outer surface of GBR procedures over top the collagen barrier membranes. There are two reasons for this—a) if PRF is left exposed to the oral cavity, its high quantity of pathogen-fighting leukocytes dramatically reduces the chance of infection (nearly tenfold); b) PRF is known to rapidly promote greater soft-tissue wound healing compared to hard tissues [11].

During the last decade, many articles focused on freeze-dried platelet products, including PRF membrane. It was reported that the new bone formation in the fresh/lyophilized PRF (1:1) was much more than that of other groups both 6 and 12 weeks in rabbits. The data suggested that growth factor concentration and release kinetics are a consequence of fresh and lyophilized PRF combination, which is an effective way to promote bone regeneration [26].

Lyophilization offers storage and processing benefits over conventional methods including longer storage time at room temperature and rapid transformation by rehydration that enables the practical application in emergency medicine and increased stability for transport. The combination of platelet-rich products and biomaterials has increased the therapeutic value of this biomaterial. PRF can bridge the gap between scaffolds and cell biology, adding the biological stimulus required for functional tissue regeneration [27].

According to some reports, freeze-drying of platelets can provide promising results and enhance the properties of the PRF membrane. Freeze-dried PRFs express their growth factors more slowly than intact ones. They have a favorable effect on bone morphogenesis and these platelets cause elevated Runt-related transcription factor 2 (Runx2) in alveolar bone and a 10-fold rise of alkaline phosphatase levels and mineralization factors. A 1.6-fold increase in osteoblast proliferation was also reported when compared to fresh PRF. A total of 97% bony coverage was detected in a rat craniofacial defect model compared to 84% for fresh PRF. The cell viability of the PRF membrane is not such an important issue in long-term bone tissue regeneration. Freeze-dried PRF, as a biomimetic scaffold without living cells, showed better biological properties in osteoblast and mesenchymal stem cell colonization and proliferation *in vitro* and animal studies as well. The possible explanations for this surprising phenomenon are increased pore size in freeze-dried PRF, which provides an ideal condition for cell adhesion and improved release of intact growth factors and cytokines [28]. Freeze-dried platelets had a five-fold increase in blood vessel density in a healing wound model with diabetic mice in contrast to the nontreated group [29].

The strengths and limitations of lyophilized platelets were collected in **Table 1**.

In spite of many articles in this field, our knowledge is still not consistent enough. There are some uncertainties due to graft properties, for example, platelet number, etc., so the processes can be standardized but the products cannot.

These membranes are prepared in centrifuge tubes alone or with metal kits. In spite of a large amount of research on this, a routine significant amount of important information is still missing that concerns the ideal preparation of the product in daily practice.

An "ideal" barrier membrane should present the following characteristics [5, 31].

- biocompatibility (to prevent adverse reactions with the surrounding tissue and with the organism);

- tissue integration (to favor the embedding in the surrounding tissue and allowing a progressive integration of collagen fibers);

- dimensional stability (the positioning and shape of the membrane should remain unaltered till degradation);

Strength
1. Preservation of biological properties
2. Preservation of morphological architecture
3. Sustained release of growth factors
4. 100% natural and autologous
5. Biocompatible with other biomaterials
6. Multiple usages with single venipuncture
7. Easy transportation
8. Better storage capabilities
9. Enables use in emergency surgery
10. Longer clinical shelf-life
Limitations
1. Fabrication cost
2. Possible risk of contamination
3. Demands standardization protocol for lyophilization technique.

Table 1.
Strengths and limitations of the lyophilized platelet concentrate (LPC) [27, 30].

- handling (the membrane should be managed and easily placed over the defect);
- selective permeability (the membrane should be able to exclude unwanted epithelial cells while allowing osteogenic cells to proliferate);
- space making function (to provide space for a stable blood clot, to allow bone regeneration).

The goal of the report is to characterize some properties of the newly invented freeze-dried human collagen membrane made of cortical bone termed SB and folded platelet-rich fibrin (F-PRF) membranes after thermal manipulation and freeze-drying. Subsequent enzymatic digestion in cell culture conditions mimics the rigor of clinical conditions. Additionally, the resistance of collagen and PRF membranes was compared.

2. Materials and methods

2.1 Preparation of collagen membrane from human cortical bone (patent pending SB by the Hisztolabor Ltd and Dent-Art-Technik, Győr, Hungary)

A 28-years old tissue donor's femoral diaphysis was processed. Cortical plates with a size of 15 × 10 × 0.5 mm were cut using a buzz saw with a diamond edge. Ten cortical plates were processed using typical bone processing, which includes defatting, decellularization, and partial decalcification. The membranes were freeze-dried in a ScanVac Superior Pro freeze-dryer (Labogene, Denmark).

2.2 Folded and non-folded PRF membrane preparation

a. **Blood collection**: blood samples were collected with the informed consent of three donors. Experiments were in accordance with the ethical standards and approval of the Regional Research and Ethics Committee. Whole blood was drawn by venipuncture from cubital veins into 36 nine-ml vacutainer tubes without any chemicals (Vacuette, Gerner BioOne).

b. **Cell separation**: due to the short lifespan of some cytokines, growth factors, and clotting of the blood sample, cell separation had to start as soon as possible, within 2 minutes maximum as previously reported [20]. Cell separation was performed by Steinberg centrifuge (CGOLDENWALL 80–2) at 375 revolutions per minute (RPM) for 10 minutes to prepare F-PRF. ~4 ml of plasma could be removed from each tube, and 16–18 ml plasma was put into eight rectangular metal jars manufactured for PRF (Dent-Art-Technik Ltd., Győr, Hungary). After 8 min at room temperature, fibrin filaments started to appear.

c. **Folded PRF preparation**: in four PRF jars in the early gelatinous stage the membrane was folded 4–5 times with forceps by seizing the corners of the membrane to completely enmesh and entrap the blood cells within the dense fibrin network (see **Figure 2a**). The membrane could be formed into different shapes by squeezing out the fluids present in the fibrin clot using a stainless steel compression device. The membranes were cut into uniform pieces and weighed.

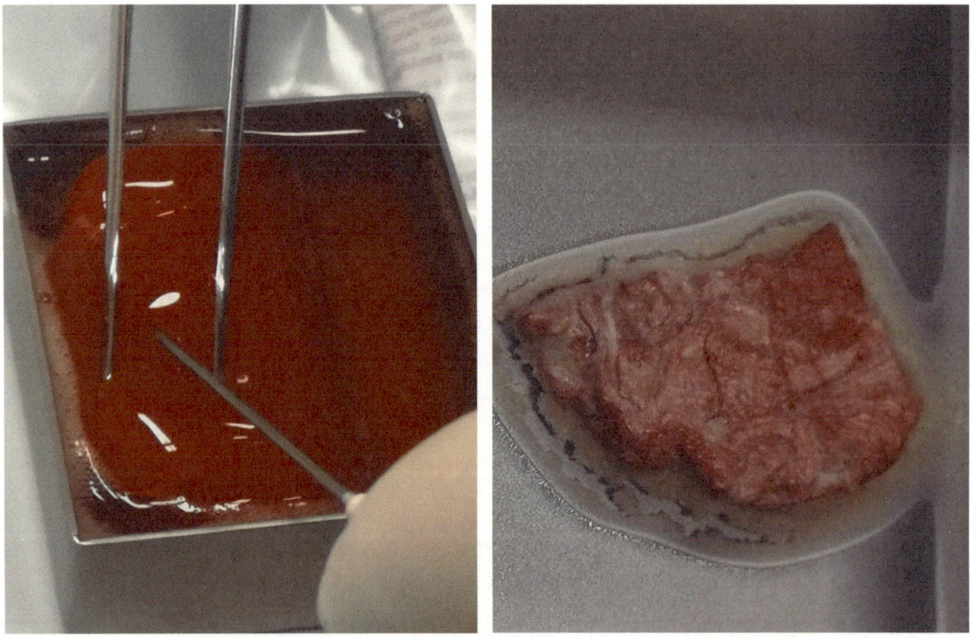

Figure 2.
(a) Preparation of folded PRF and (b) freeze-dried F-PRF. Note cracked surfaces.

d. **Unfolded, intact PRF preparation**: in four PRF jars the plasma was left intact until there was clotting and spontaneous formation of the flat rectangular membrane. The membranes were cut into uniform pieces and weighed.

2.3 Freeze-drying of F-PRF membranes

The same procedure was performed as in the SB membrane (see #2.1 and **Figure 2B**).

2.4 Determination of moisture content after FD by gravimetry

Samples of freeze-dried F-PRF and SB collagen membrane (five pieces from each group) were put into a drying chamber (Binder, Germany) for 1 h at 90°C to remove the remnant moisture of lyophilized tissue and assess the efficacy of FD. The tissue samples were weighed after freeze-drying and heat drying as well.

2.5 Rehydration

All membrane pieces of the three groups (SB collagen membrane, folded PRF, and intact PRF) were put in rehydration fluid. Half of them were submerged into a PS, the other half were rehydrated in the blood donor's serum. According to a previous experiment during 10 min of rehydration, all the membranes were saturated with moisture and their weight did not change over the next 20 min of rehydration.

After freeze-drying, the pieces were weighed. According to our previous report, the F-PRF is superior to a conventional non-folded membrane, so only fresh and lyophilized rehydrated F-PRF and lyophilized SB membrane were investigated in the following #6 experiment [20]. Unpaired two-sample t-tests were performed to compare the differences of the relevant experimental groups.

2.6 Membrane resistance against proteolytic digestion

The objective of this experiment was to mimic the clinical conditions and assess the resistance of membranes against enzymatic protein digestion after transplantation. Three groups (freeze-dried SB collagen, freeze-dried and rehydrated F-PRF, fresh F-PRF) were prepared by cutting them into uniform pieces. All fresh, freeze-dried and rehydrated membranes were weighed then kept in Dulbecco's minimal essential medium (DMEM) containing 0.1% (v/v) trypsin (Sigma, USA) and 0.4 mg/ml EDTA (ethylene diamine tetraacetic acid) at cell culture conditions in a HeraCell 150 CO_2 thermostat (Heraeus, Germany) at +37°C in 5% CO_2 to feed the membranes. DMEM with trypsin was replaced every day. The weights of membrane pieces were assessed every 24 h using a laboratory scale (Kern, Germany) for 21 days. The samples were kept in a 2-ml mixture in a 24 cell well plate.

2.7 Histology

HE, trichrome, and immunohistological staining (VEGF) were performed in the fresh F-PRF and the SB groups.

3. Results

The results of thermal manipulations can be seen in **Table 2**. The SB membrane lost more than 50% weight during FD. The folded PRF membrane lost less water than the non-folded membrane in percentage, and both membranes became fragile after freeze-drying (see **Figure 2b**).

The difference between the rehydration capacity of folded and non-folded PRF membranes is significant ($p < 0.01$). No difference was found between PS and blood serum after rehydration. The SB membrane regained 66% of the original weight (see **Table 2**).

Weight after freeze drying			
Folded PRF (n = 15)	16.2 ± 2.2%		
Non folded PRF (n = 15)	10.3 ± 4.1%		
SB (n = 10)	43 ± 0.4%		
Weight after rehydration (10 min)			
F-PRF		**Non folded PRF**	
PS (n = 5)	serum (n = 5)	PS (n = 5)	serum (n = 5)
52.4 ± 4.8%	48.4 ± 2.4%	30 ± 6.8%	30.8 ± 7.2%
SB (n = 5; in PS only): 66 ± 0.3%			
Moisture remnant after freeze-drying:			
F-PRF (n = 5): 3.2 ± 0.3%			
Non folded-PRF (n = 5): 3.3 ± 0.3%			
SB (n = 5): 3.9 ± 0.4%			

Table 2.
Comparison of weights after freeze drying and rehydration process. The original fresh weight of the PRF membranes was set at 100%. The processed decalcified weight was set at 100% in SB. (PS-physiological salt solution).

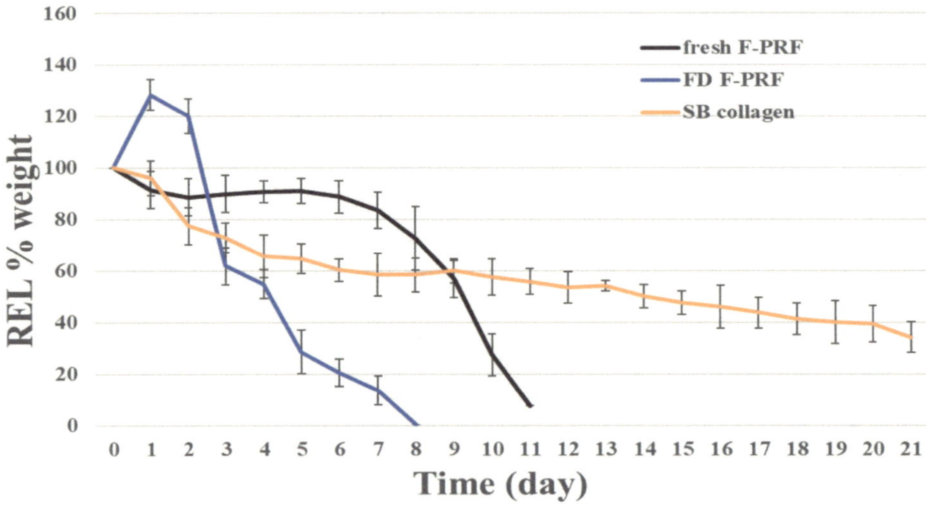

Figure 3.
Proteolytic digestion in membranes. Weights were expressed in relative %. On day 0 the rehydrated weight was set at 100% in freeze-dried PRF and SB membranes. Bars are standard deviations.

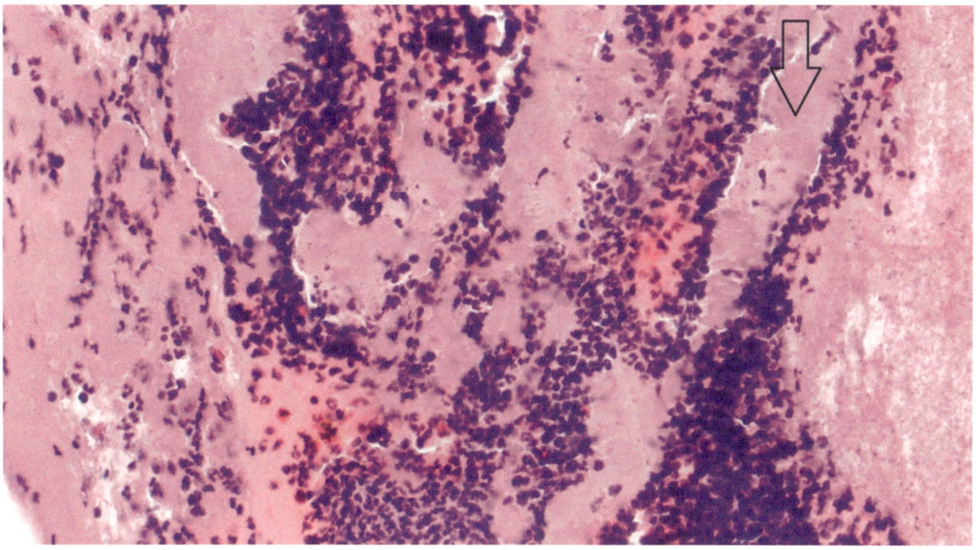

Figure 4.
Histology of fresh F-PRF membrane (HE, 400× magnification). In a fresh F-PRF membrane remarkable cell quantity can be seen. There are big leukocyte groups separated by fibrin bunches (arrow).

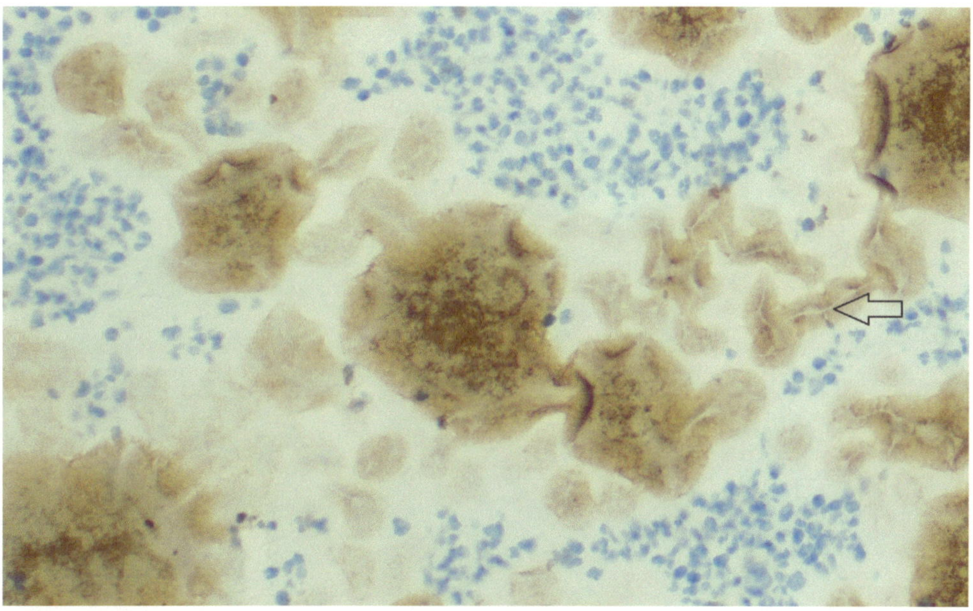

Figure 5.
Cloudy brown VEGF (vascular endothelial growth factor) positivity can be seen around dense platelet groups (VEGF immunohistology, 400× magnification). Blue cells are leukocytes. Note the remarkable early phase of vasculogenesis (arrow), which is a key issue in tissue morphogenesis.

The moisture content was under 5% in both PRF groups and in SB as well after FD.

There was a remarkable resistance against enzymatic digestion for 1 week in fresh F-PRF. During the 2nd week, dissolving was accelerated. The fresh F-PRF was

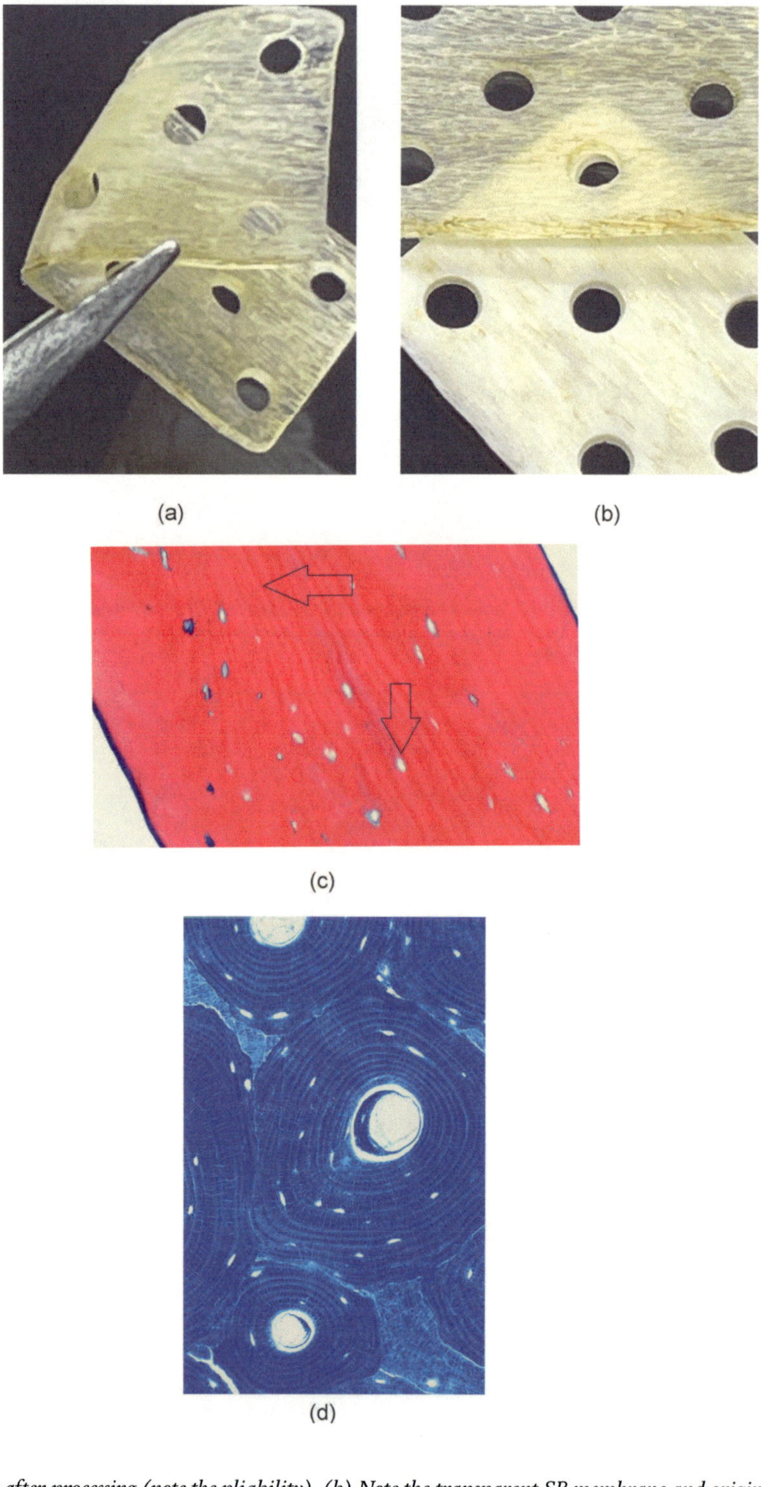

Figure 6.
(a) SoftBone after processing (note the pliability). (b) Note the transparent SB membrane and original intact cortical bone plate with holes. (c) Histology: parallel red collagen fibers can be seen in decalcified SB (horizontal arrow). The osteocyte lacuna is empty (vertical arrow). (trichrome staining 400×). (d) SB membrane after 3 weeks of enzymatic digestion. The original osteon units of cortical bone can still be recognized with central Haversian canals. (Trichrome staining 400×).

obviously superior to the freeze-dried F-PRF, which disintegrated on the 8th day. The SB collagen membrane had the best resistance. Until the 21st day, it preserved 34% of the original rehydrated weight (see **Figure 3**).

Histology and immunohistology: the F-PRF contains many cells in homogenous distribution, especially leukocytes and platelets in a dense fibrin network (**Figure 4**).

The SB membrane became pliable and transparent after tissue processing, freeze-drying, and rehydration (see **Figure 6a** and **b**). In decalcified and processed bone the collagen was preserved (see **Figure 6c**). After 3 weeks of enzymatic digestion in spite of remarkable weight loss, the original structure seemed to be intact. The blue color is a sign of molecular tissue disintegration using the same trichrome staining (see **Figure 6d**).

4. Discussion

During freeze-drying, the F-PRF lost less moisture in comparison to the non-folded one (84% vs. 90%). Squeezing removes more serum in F-PRF than in the spontaneous contraction of fibrin network in non-folded PRF membrane, so the latter had higher initial water content.

After rehydration, the F-PRF could regain more than half of its original weight, while intact PRF reached only 30%. It seems that the folding technique provides advantages in this field too; probably the water binding capacity remained more intact this way. Ten minutes are enough for rehydration, but freeze-dried PRF membrane could absorb almost 30% more additional moisture slowly during the next 24 h (see **Figure 3**).

There was no significant difference between the PS and blood serum as a rehydrant. The folded and non-folded PRF membranes were rehydrated by solution in the same manner. SB became pliable again after rehydration, so it can be adapted to irregular surfaces.

The SB collagen membrane showed more resistant properties in tissue culture conditions than the F-PRF membrane. The freeze-dried F-PRF could not withstand the double rigor of tissue culture conditions and enzymatic digestion that mimic the *in vivo* clinical conditions in the oral cavity. The membranes are separated from saliva and oral liquids clinically in optimal conditions, but they are exposed to long-term unfavorable enzymatic and protecting cellular effects. The fresh F-PRF disintegrated after 11 days and the freeze-dried F-PRF membranes dissolved on the 8th day in these conditions. After 3 weeks of storage, the SB membrane still seemed intact macroscopically but its weight fell to 34% of its original.

It seems the folding procedure increases the resistance and density of the fibrin network serving as a biological autoscaffold and showed better resistance against enzymatic digestion of membrane proteins in fresh F-PRF. In contrast to the fresh membrane, freeze-drying decreased the resistance of the F-PRF membrane so its disintegration was faster.

The biological value of fresh F-PRF membranes is remarkable in that it contains homogenously distributed active living cells. The early phase of vasculogenesis can be found after few minutes, which is very astounding and an important milestone on the path to developing blood supply in tissue morphogenesis (see **Figures 4** and **5**).

The F-PRF process obviously requires manual manipulation, so it needs to be performed under aseptic conditions clinically. After the early introduction of open-system experts were alerted to safety issues [32]. During the last decade, the huge and emerging number of clinical cases did not confirm the worries. There were no available references on serious adverse events (SAE) or serious adverse reactions (SAR) in regard to the application of platelet and leukocyte-rich products.

Freeze-drying as a preservation method can produce well manageable tissue samples and even enhance some favorable properties of PRF.

The resorbable collagen membranes, including SB, do not have such an attractive biological value but they do have their advantages. They serve like a natural protective biological scaffold for tissue morphogenesis. SoftBone is an allogeneic decellularized and decalcified flexible bone membrane, which mostly consists of collagen type I. It provides an optimal condition for host cells to potentially have ideal pore sizes. Its remarkable resistance against enzymatic digestion *in vitro* makes it a good choice alone or in combination with PRF membrane for long-term protection of grafted bone; however, further studies are required to find the optimal membrane type for GBR.

5. Conclusion

Resorbable barrier membranes, including platelet-rich fibrin (PRF) and collagen membranes, can play a key role in guided bone regeneration surgeries (GBR) in dentistry. PRF membranes have a high biological value containing a lot of cytokines and growth factors. In spite of good reported experimental results of freeze-dried PRF, its enzymatic disintegration was faster than in fresh PRF. SoftBone membrane made of partially decalcified allogeneic cortical bone can be easily adapted to diverse surfaces and showed satisfying resistance against proteolytic trypsin digestion. Further studies will show the long-term fate of SB membrane in animal and clinical studies.

F-PRF and SB membranes alone or in combination have an excellent potential to become ideal membranes in GBR.

Acknowledgements

We would like to express our thanks to Mr. John Kowalchuk for his support in editing the manuscript.

Abbreviations

FD	freeze-drying (lyophilization)
F-PRF	folded platelet-rich fibrin
GBR	guided bone regeneration
HE	hematoxylin–eosin staining
PRF	platelet-rich fibrin
PS	physiological salt solution
SB	SoftBone membrane (patent pending product)
VEGF	vascular endothelial growth factor

Author details

Lajos Csönge[1*], Ágnes Bozsik[1], Zoltán T. Bagi[2], Róbert Gyuris[3], Dóra K. Csönge[4] and János Kónya[5]

1 West Hungarian Regional Tissue Bank, Petz A. University Teaching Hospital, Győr, Hungary

2 Private Practice, Budapest, Hungary

3 Private Practice, Eger, Hungary

4 Pepperdine University, Malibu, CA, United States

5 Dent-Art-Technik Ltd., Győr and Széchenyi University, Győr, Hungary

*Address all correspondence to: luisbathhelena@gmail.com

References

[1] LeHuec JC, Sadikki R, Cogniet A, et al. Role of a collagen membrane in adhesion prevention strategy for complex spinal surgeries. International Orthopaedics (SICOT). 2015;**39**:1383-1390. DOI: 10.1007/s00264-015-2767-x

[2] Dabrowski A, Lepère M, Zaranis C, Coelio C, Hauters P. Efficacy and safety of a resorbable collagen membrane COVA+ for the prevention of postoperative adhesions in abdominal surgery. Surgical Endoscopy. 2016;**30**(6): 2358-2366. DOI: 10.1007/s00464-015-4484-3. Epub 2015 Oct 19. PMID: 26482156

[3] Theys T, Van Hoylandt A, Broeckx CE, Van Gerven L. Plasma-rich fibrin in neurosurgery: A feasibility study. Acta Neurochirurgica. 2018;**160**(8):1497-1503. DOI: 10.1007/s00701-018-3579-8

[4] Dawood AS, Salem HA. Current clinical applications of platelet-rich plasma in various gynecological disorders: An appraisal of theory and practice. Clinical and Experimental Reproductive Medicine. 2018;**45**(2):67-74. DOI: 10.5653/cerm.2018.45.2.67

[5] Sbricoli L, Guazzo R, Annunziata M, Gobbato L, Bressan E, Nastri L. Selection of collagen membranes for bone regeneration: A literature review. Materials (Basel). 2020;**13**(3):786. DOI: 10.3390/ma13030786

[6] Available from: https://www.zimmerbiometdental.com/content/dam/zb-dental/products/clinical-summaries/zb0792_rev_a_in_vitro_degradation_collagen-based_membranes_clinical_poster_final_secured.pdf

[7] Kolerman R, Qahaz N, Barnea E, Mijiritsky E, Chaushu L, Tal H, et al. Allograft and collagen membrane augmentation procedures preserve the bone level around implants after immediate placement and restoration. International Journal of Environmental Research and Public Health. 2020;**17**(4):1133. DOI: 10.3390/ijerph17041133

[8] Choukroun J, Diss A, Simonpieri A, Marie-Odile Girard MO, et al. Platelet-rich fibrin (PRF): A second-generation platelet concentrate. Part IV: Clinical effects on tissue healing. Oral Surgery, Oral Medicine, Oral Pathology, Oral Radiology, and Endodontics. 2006;**101**(3):e56-e60. DOI: 10.1016/j.tripleo.2005.07.011

[9] Marx RE, Carlson ER, Eichstaedt RM, Schimmele SR, Strauss JE, Georgeff KR. Platelet-rich plasma: Growth factor enhancement for bone grafts. Oral Surgery, Oral Medicine, Oral Pathology, Oral Radiology, and Endodontics. 1998;**85**(6):638-646. DOI: 10.1016/s1079-2104(98)90029-4

[10] Borie E, Olivi DG, Orsi IA, et al. Platelet-rich fibrin application in dentistry: A literature review. International Journal of Clinical and Experimental Medicine. 2015;**8**(5):7922-7929

[11] Miron RJ, Pikos MA. PRF as a Barrier Membrane in Guided Bone Regeneration. 2018. Available from: https://www.dentalcetoday.com/wp-content/uploads/2018/06/1217_Miron_CE_216.pdf

[12] Everts PAM et al. Platelet-rich plasma and platelet gel: A review the conventional way of PRF membrane preparation is the cell separation and serum squeezing. The Journal of The American Society of Extra-Corporeal Technology. 2006;**38**:174-187

[13] Chaparro O, Linero I. Regenerative medicine: A new paradigm in bone regeneration. In: Advanced Techniques in Bone Regeneration. Chapter 12. IntechOpen. 2016. pp. 253-274. DOI: 10.5772/62523

[14] Crisci A, Manfred S, Crisci M. The L-PRF membrane (fibrin rich in platelets and leukocytes) and its derivatives useful as a source of stem cells in wound surgery. Journal of Stem Cell Reports. 2019;**1**:1-11

[15] Kemmochi M, Sasaki S, Takahashi M, Nishimura T, Aizawa C, Kikuchi J. The use of platelet-rich fibrin with platelet plasma support meniscal repair surgery. Journal of Orthopaedics. 2018;**15**:711-720

[16] Fujioka Kobayashi M, Schaller B, Mourao CFDAB, et al. Biological characterization of an injectable platelet-rich fibrin mixture consisting of autologous albumin gel and liquid platelet-rich fibrin (Alb-PRF). Platelets. 2020;**20**:1-8. DOI: 10.1080/09537104.2020.1717455

[17] Ehrenfest DMD, Pinto NR, Pereda A, et al. The impact of the centrifuge charasteristics and centrifugation protocols on the cells, growth factors, and fibrin architecture of leukocyte-and platelet-rich fibrin (L-PRF) clot and membrane. Platelets. 2018;**29**(2):171-184

[18] Takahashi A, Tsujino T, Yamaguchi S, et al. Distrubution of platelets, transforming growth factor-β1, platelet-derived growth factor-BB, vascular endothelial growth factor and matrix metalloprotease-9 in advanced platelet-rich fibrin and concentrated growth factor matrices. Journal of Investigative and Clinical Dentistry. 2019;**10**(4):00e12458. DOI: 10.1111/jicd.12458

[19] Isobe K, Watanebe T, Kawabata H, et al. Mechanical and degradation properties of advanced platelet-rich fibrin (A-PRF), concentrated growth factors (CGF), and platelet-poor plasma-derived fibrin (PPTF). International Journal of Implant Dentistry. 2017;**1**:17. DOI: 10.1186/s40729-017-0081-7

[20] Csönge L, Bozsik Á, Tóth-Bagi Z, Gyuris R, Kónya J. Regenerative medicine: Characterization of human bone matrix gelatin (BMG) and folded platelet-rich fibrin (F-PRF) membranes alone and in combination (sticky bone). Cell and Tissue Banking. 2021;**22**:711-717. DOI: 10.1007/s10561-021-09925-9

[21] Kardos D, Hornyák I, Simon M, et al. Biological and mechanical properties of platelet-rich fibrin membrane after thermal manipulation and preparation in a single-syringe closed system. International Journal of Molecular Sciences. 2018;**19**(11):3433. DOI: 10.3390/ijms19113433

[22] Ehrenfest DM, Diss A, Odin G, Doglioli P, Hippolyte M-P, Charrier J-B. In vitro effects of Choukroun's PRF (platelet-rich fibrin) on human gingival fibroblasts, dermal prekeratinocytes, preadipocytes, and maxillofacial osteoblasts in primary cultures. Oral Surgery, Oral Medicine, Oral Pathology, Oral Radiology, and Endodontics. 2009;**108**:341-352. [CrossRef]

[23] Yung Y-L, Fu S-C, Cheuk Y-C, Qin L, Ong MT-Y, Chan K-M, et al. Optimisation of platelet concentrates therapy:Composition, localisation, and duration of action. Asia-Pacific Journal of Sports Medicine Arthroscopic Rehabilitation Technology. 2017;7:27-36

[24] Abdullah MO, Hayder AA. Collagen membrane versus platelet rich fibrin membrane in bone graft healing:

An experimental study in sheep. EDJ. 2020;**3**(2):104-111. DOI: 10.15218/edj.2020.15

[25] Gassling V, Hedderich J, Açil Y, Purcz N, Wiltfang J, Douglas T. Comparison of platelet rich fibrin and collagen as osteoblast-seeded scaffolds for bone tissue engineering applications. Clinical Oral Implants Research. 2011;**00**(2011):1-9. DOI: 10.1111/j.1600-0501.2011.02333.x

[26] Liu Z, Jin H, Xie Q, Jiang Z, Guo S, Li Y, et al. Controlled release strategies for the combination of fresh and lyophilized platelet-rich fibrin on bone tissue regeneration. Hindawi BioMed Research International. 2019;**10**: Article ID 4923767. DOI: 10.1155/2019/4923767

[27] Ngah NA, Ratnayake J, Cooper PR, Dias GJ, Tong DC, Mohd Noor SNF, et al. Potential of lyophilized platelet concentrates for craniofacial tissue regenerative therapies. Molecules. 2021;**26**:517. DOI: 10.3390/molecules26030517

[28] Li Q, Reed DA, Min L, Gopinathan G, Li S, et al. Lyophilized platelet-rich fibrin (PRF) promotes craniofacial bone regeneration through Runx2. International Journal of Molecular Sciences. 2014;**15**:8509-8525. DOI: 10.3390/ijms15058509

[29] Pietramaggiori G, Kaipainen A, Czeczuga JM, Christopher TW, Orgill DP. Freeze-dried platelet-rich plasma shows beneficial healing properties in chronic wounds. Wound Repair and Regeneration. 2006;**14**:573-580

[30] Andia I, Perez-Valle A, Del Amo C, Maffulli N. Freeze-drying of platelet-rich plasma: The quest for standardization. International Journal of Molecular Sciences. 2020;**21**:6904

[31] Calciolari E, Ravanetti F, Strange A, Mardas N, Bozec L, Cacchioli A, et al. Degradation pattern of a porcine collagen membrane in an in vivo model of guided bone regeneration. Journal of Periodontal Research. 2018;**53**:430-439

[32] O'Connell SM. Safety issues associated with platelet-rich fibrin. Method letters to the editor. Oral Radiology Endodontics. 2007;**5**:587

Section 2

Tissue Engineering

Chapter 5

Collagen-Based Biomaterial as Drug Delivery Module

Amit Kumar Verma

Abstract

In the field of medicine, controlled drug delivery has become a major challenge due to inefficiency of drug at critical parameters such as permeability, solubility, half-life, targeting ability, bio- & hemocompatibility, immunogenicity, off-target toxicity and biodegradability. Since several decades the role of drug delivery module has been a crucial parameter of research and clinical observations to improve the effectiveness of drugs. Biomaterials- natural or artificial are mainly used for medical application such as in therapeutics or in diagnostics. Among all the biomaterials, collagen based-hydrogels/ films/ composite materials have attracted the research and innovations and are the excellent objects for drug delivery, tissue engineering, wound dressings and gene therapeutics etc. due to high encapsulating capacity, mechanically strong swollen structural network and efficient mass transfer properties. Substantial developments have been performed using collagen-based drug delivery systems (DDS) to deliver biomolecules with better efficacy. In spite of significant progress, several issues at clinical trials particularly targeting of intracellular molecules such as genes is still a challenge for researchers. Experimental results, theoretical models, molecular simulations will boost the fabrication/ designing of collage-based DDS, which further will enhance the understanding of controlled delivery/mechanism of therapeutics at specific targets for various disease treatments.

Keywords: collagen, biomaterial, drug delivery systems (DDS), drug, hydrogels, films, composite material

1. Introduction

Collagen is unique and major structural protein of extracellular matrix (ECM) and plays crucial role to the structural integrity of tissues/organs and cellular growth in vertebrates and other organisms, constitute around 30% of the total protein content of mammal's body, involved in mechanical protection of tissues and organs such as skin, tendons, ligaments, bones, cartilage, blood vessels, cornea and nails etc. (**Figure 1**) [1–6]. More than 50% in the skin and more than 90% of extracellular proteins in the tendon and bone is made up of collagen [7, 8].

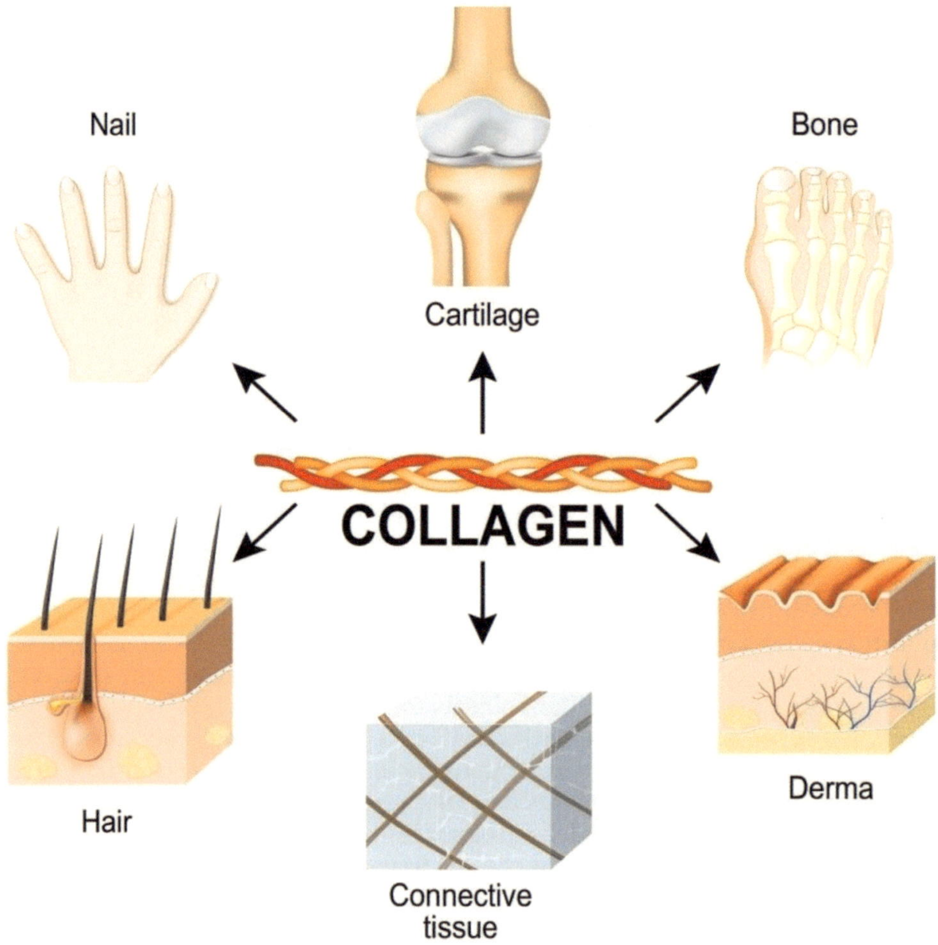

Figure 1.
Collagen's occurrence in different body tissues.

The unique feature of collagen molecule is triple helix structure made by three identical or non-identical polypeptide chains. Each polypeptide chain comprises around 1000 amino acids and the chains are supercoiled in left handed manner around the axis with staggering of residues between adjacent chains, give rise to triple helix right handed structure [9]. Each chain is having the repeated sequence of (Gly-X-Y)*n*, whereas X and Y are mostly proline and hydroxyproline residues [1, 10, 11]. At present, 30 different types of collagens have been characterized and reported in literature [12]. Among all the different variants of collagen, type I, II, III, V and XI represent more than 90% of human fibrillar collagen and is majorly distributed in dermis, hair, bone, cartilage, ligament, tendon and placenta [13]. Other types such as type IV and VIII form the network frame of basement membranes [12, 14]. Type I collagen has very important role in medicine as well as in development of medical devices, artificial implants, drug carriers for controlled release and scaffolds for tissue regeneration [5, 15, 16]. Being the highly versatile, structurally unique and biocompatible protein substance, the collagen can be developed into different types of drug/active substance carrier module such as hydrogels, microparticles and films etc. [3, 7].

2. Collagen as a biomaterial

According to Hench and Erthridge, 1982 [17], "a biomaterial is used to make devices to replace a part or a function of the body in a safe, reliable, economic, and physiologically acceptable manner." Raghavendra et al. [18] has mentioned the other definitions of biomaterial are "materials of synthetic as well as of natural origin in contact with tissue, blood, and biological fluids, intended for use for prosthetic, diagnostic, therapeutic, and storage applications without adversely affecting the living organism and its components" [19] and "any substance (other than drugs) or combination of substances, synthetic or natural in origin, which can be used for any period of time, as a whole or as a part of a system which treats, augments, or replaces any tissue, organ, or function of the body" [20]. Application of biomaterials in physiological systems is possible due to competent and stable features of biomaterials [21] which can be achieved with proper combination of mechanical, physical, chemical and biological attributes [22]. Modern biomaterials are designed and developed singly or in combinations of polymers, metals, composite materials and ceramics etc. [18].

In the field of medicine, collagen is one of the most studied biomaterial or biopolymer and according to Cheng et al. [23], around 260,000 literature articles (at present, the number is many more than reported) reported it as pivotal component in tissue regeneration and so called as 'the steel of the biological material". Collagen is the main biopolymer of ECM of vertebrates and invertebrates and has the capability to interact with large number of biomolecules leading to various biological reactions/changes under normal or pathological processes in the body, inspiring the scientists to develop the various formulations based on collagen [24–26]. The attributes for the testimony of collagen's usage in wide scenario of medicine are its cosmopolitanism, high biocompatibility, hemocompatibility, biomimetic and biodegradability and to make composite biopolymer with biomaterials like chitosan (CHS), alginate (ALG), cellulose (CL), hyaluronic acid (HA), glycosaminoglycans (GAGs) as well as synthetic materials like carboxy methyl cellulose (CMC), poly vinyl alcohol (PVA), poly ε-caprolactone (PCL), poly ethyl methacrylate (PEMA) etc. in different formulations [27–29].

Now it is well established that collagen has good elasticity, physical, mechanical, enzymatic and thermal stability inside the body environment, but after extraction and utilization these properties are compromised at large scale [30–32], so the additional need of chemicals, chemical and physical processes are required to develop the stable biomaterial. Though extracted collagen is a promising drug delivery material in the field of ophthalmology but can be easily degradable *in vitro* due to disruption of natural intermolecular crosslinks of lysine and hydroxylysine residues during isolation and purification process [33]. The weaknesses of extracted collagen such as mechanical and thermal strength, enzymatic degradation can be reduced with the help of various methods of chemical, physical and enzymatic crosslinking, covalent conjugating, grafting polymerization or blending. The blended collagen-based biomaterials like hydrogels, films, microspheres and nanoparticles (NPs) have low immunogenicity, good absorption, hemostatic property and synergism with other bioactive compounds or loaded drugs and remain unaltered after several processes. The requirement of mechanical, pH, enzymatic, thermal stability is not provided alone by collagen for a controlled DDS but can be achieved with combination of CHS or ALG for release of analgesics, chemotherapeutic molecules and natural bioactive agent like curcumin or aloe vera. The blended biopolymer will have the combined desired properties of the separate material. Hydrogel of blended collagen-CHS have antibacterial, antifungal, anti-carcinogenic and immunogenic attributes [34–37]. Blended collagen-CL based

Biopolymers	Source	Stability	Toxicity	Biomedical property	Applications	References
Collagen	Vertebrate protein (skin, bone, tendon, dentin, cornea, cartilage, vessels, intestine, uterus, dermis, placenta	Poor mechanical, thermal, enzymatic, tensile rigidity	Insignificant	Biocompatible, biomimetic fibril forming, self-assembling, biodegradable	Food, cosmetics, ophthalmology, inserts, shields, particles, gels, aqueous injectables, drug delivery, Grafting, tissue engineering	[38, 40, 42–44]
Alginate	Brown algae (Phaeophyceae family), *Laminaria hyperborea*, *Laminaria digitata*, *Laminaria japonica*, *Ascophyllum nodosum* & *Macrocystis pyrifera*	Poor mechanical and chemical	Low	Biocompatibiliy, mild gelation	Wound healing, delivery of bioactive agents like small drugs, proteins, tissue engineering, cell transplantation	[45–48]
Chitosan	From chitin of insects, crustaceans, cephalopods cephalopods	Mechanically strong	Insignificant	Nontoxic, non-immunogenic, non-immunogenic, non-carcinogenic, biocompatible, bioabsorbable, antimicrobial, antifungal, anticoagulant, anti-tumor, hemostatic	Biosensors, drug delivery, wound dressing	[35, 49–51]
Cellulose	Wood, cotton, sugarbeet potato, tubers, onion, hemp, flax, wheat straw, mulberry bark, algae, bacteria	Mechanically high	Insignificant	Biocompatible, biodegradable, biological affinity, antibacterial	Wound dressing, shields, dental implants, bone tissue grafting, artificial blood vessel	[37, 52–54]

Table 1.
Natural and abundant biopolymers: Sources, properties, and potential applications.

hydrogel has properties like biomimetic and hemostatic from collagen while mechanical strength and antibacterial characteristic from CL. In the field of ophthalmology blended collagen-based hydrogels with CHS or ALG are applied for corneal disease treatment exhibiting good mechanical and thermal attributes along with transparency. The films, microspheres, membranes and scaffolds of blended collagen-based materials are used in wound dressing due to moisture retaining, low adhesion, absorption of blood and tissue exudates, anti-infective and permeability properties [32, 38–41]. The sources and possible applications of most utilized material of blended biopolymers along with important features like stability, toxicity and biomedical are presented in **Table 1**.

3. Crosslinking for collagen-based biomaterial

Collagen is the most abundant vertebrate protein and mostly used biopolymer and with variety of physiological features like biocompatible, low immunogenic, self assembling fibril formation etc. The collagen is mechanically strong and durable *in vivo* but after the isolation and purification processes is vulnerable to degradation *in vitro* due to dissociation of natural crosslinks and assembly structure by neutral salt, acid alkali or proteases and quality of extracted collagen is inferior to native state (**Figure 2**) [42, 55]. The researchers are attempting to make the suitable collagen-based biomaterial with properties of increased mechanical strength, reduced enzymatic degradation, stability, solubility and low toxicity by introducing exogenous crosslinking [42, 56]. The introduced intermolecular crosslinking prevents the unknotting of collagen fibrils produced by heat and advancing the thermal stability along with increased tensile strength, stiffness, compressive modulus and decreased extensibility [57–60]. The exogenous natural or chemical crosslinks could significantly reduce the enzymatic degradation of collagen by blocking the cleavage site [61].

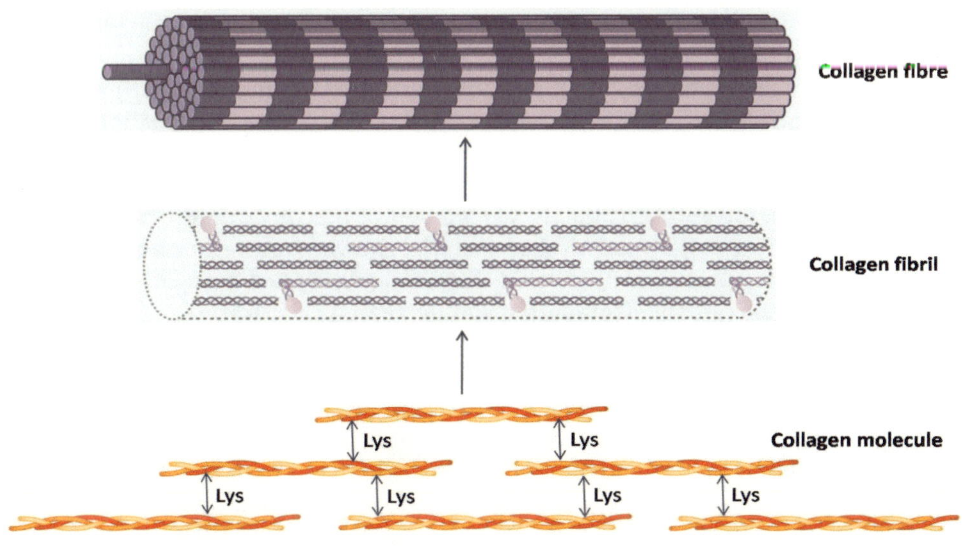

Figure 2.
Native crosslinking in the collagen molecules.

Though collagen-based crosslinked biopolymers are producing significant results in the field of biomedicine and biotechnology, still no standard method is applicable to the formulation of improved non-toxic and biocompatible hydrogels, films and matrices etc. Different crosslinking strategies such as chemical, physical or enzymatic are applied to achieve the collagen-based materials with desired properties for drug delivery and other applications [62].

3.1 Chemical crosslinking

The most used crosslinking method is with chemical agents due to ease of application, less time consuming and cost effective. The most commonly used chemical reagents are formaldehyde (FA) and glutaraldehyde (GTA). FA reacts with the ε-amino group of lysine and hydroxylysine residue of collagen to form imine as an intermediate followed by crosslink with tyrosine or with amide group of asparagine or glutamine residue. FA-crosslinked products generated brittleness, significant toxicity and unfavorable reactions, hence not preferred in biomedicine [7]. Another agent GTA is widely utilized for crosslinking of collagen, based on high reactivity and low cost. The low concentration of FA and GTA produced brittle and low uniformity of composites while high concentration led to major cytotoxic effects. Several methods have been applied to remove the unreacted GTA, due to its cytotoxicity the use of GTA at present scenario is still debatable [28, 42]. Hexa-methylene-diisocyanate (HDC) was used as an alternative to GTA, but in contrast to GTA, HDC showed less severe primary and secondary cytotoxicity during cell proliferation as compared to non-crosslinked material [63]. Charulatha & Rajaram [64] evaluated the biocompatibility of collagen membranes cross-linked with 3,3′-dithio bis-propionimidate (DTBP) and dimethyl suberimidate (DMS). Both DTBP and DMS showed lower toxicity than GTA and as the better substitute for crosslinking. The polyepoxy compounds such as ethylene glycol diglycidyl ether, glycerol polyglycidyl ether and methyl glycidyl ether were used as crosslinker [65]. The epoxy group reacts with amino group of lysine residue for crosslinking similar to GTA. The polyepoxy crosslinked material showed acceptable cytotoxicity [66].

Due to non-toxicity and water solubility, the carbodiimides and acyl azides showed significant crosslinking with collagen. Carbodiimides like 1-(3-dimethylaminopropyl)-3-ethylcarbodiimide (EDC) and N-hydroxy succinimide (NHS) are better candidate than aldehydes, HDC and polyepoxy compounds due to formation of amide bonds between –COOH and –NH_2 group of collagen without becoming the part of actual linkage. Van Wachem et al. [67] compared the four crosslinking methods i.e. GTA, HDC, acyl azide and EDC for the assessment of biocompatibility and tissue regeneration ability and EDC crosslinked material showed best results among the four tested methods. Pieper et al. [68] showed that EDC crosslinked collagen expressed no cytotoxicity, slow enzymatic degradation and decreased calcification.

Non-toxic, biodegradable and biocompatible natural compounds as promising cross-linkers like alginic acid (anionic block copolymer) from brown algae, iridoid compounds from the fruits of *Gardenia jasminoides* and *Genipa americana* [69], oxidized alginate [70], dialdehyde starch [71], D, L-glyceraldehyde [72], natural polyphenols and dialdehyde- carboxymethyl cellulose [73] have been broadly examined. In recent years usage of polyphenols such as caffeic acid (CA) and tannic acid (TA) [74], proanthocyanidin [75], procyanidin [76], epigallocatechin gallate (EGCG) and epicatechin gallates (ECG) [77] and other tannins [78] have been increased due to antioxidative, anti-inflammatory, antimicrobial, cardioprotective, antithrombotic, pharmacological and therapeutic possibilities. According to Jackson et al. [77] TA, EGCG and ECG showed stabilization of collagen implant for long period at very low concentration and protection against collagenase more effectively than GTA and carbodiimides. In contrast to GTA, natural crosslinkers have disadvantages like long term storage and degree of crosslinking.

3.2 Physcial crosslinking

Physical techniques like ionizing radiation (X-ray and γ-ray), UV light and dehydrothermal treatment and dye-mediated photo-oxidation are used as crosslinkers for collagen based formulations. The physical crosslinking relies on the factors like amount of radiation, temperature, hydration conditions, electron beam intensity and UV denaturation [43]. Photosensitizer riboflavin in combination with UV-irradiation produced the similar results of crosslinking by GTA without cytotoxicity to reduce the harmful effects of physical and chemical crosslinking [45]. UV- light mediated crosslinking generated the denaturation and conformational modifications of collagen molecules which opposed the stabilization of UV-induced crosslinked product [79]. Dehydrothermal treatment resulted into the complex of collagen with anatomically accepted structures without contraction, curling or deformity for longer duration without the involvement of chemical crosslinking [80]. In contrast to chemical crosslinking the heating disrupted the triple helical conformation of collagen and increased the degradation by enzymes [81]. Overall the physical crosslinking methods are simple and safe for the production of splendid biocompatible biomaterials in comparison to exogenous cytotoxic chemical crosslinkers.

3.3 Enzymatic crosslinking

Enzymatic approaches have gained interest due to brilliant specificity and accurate reaction kinetics and to surmount the difficulties with chemical methods. Enzymatic crosslinkers can be categorized into oxidoreductases, transferases and hydrolases based on the catalytic reaction [82]. The oxidative enzymes tyrosinase and laccase [83] along with acyltransferase-transglutaminase have the capacity to modify the protein substrate to enhance the quality of crosslinked biomaterials [84]. Transglutaminases are calcium dependent and catalyze the reactions in broad range of pH and temperatures. Microbial origin biodegradable transglutaminases can catalyze the crosslinking in the concentration dependent manner [85, 86]. Exogenous lysyl oxidase catalyzes the lysine residue into highly reactive aldehydes leading to the formation of crosslinks in the ECM proteins. The pre-treatment of lysyl oxidase promoted the maturation of native and engineered collagen tissues both *in vitro* and *in vivo* with reference to increased tensile modulus and pyridinoline crosslinking [87].

Comparing all the crosslinking strategies the chemical method is the most preferred due to generation of consistent and high degree of crosslinking [88]. The physical method is used as a appurtenant crosslinking approach. Enzymatic approach alleviates the shortcomings produced by chemical and physical crosslinking methods, but it is time consuming and expensive [89]. In recent years, the use of natural and eco-friendly biocompatible crosslinkers has increased and become the very promising agents. The natural substance- genipin obtained from irridoid glucoside (geniposide) is one of the important crosslinker with great potential in the field of biomedicine. Genipin is very expensive in contrast to other natural crosslinkers, while TA is cheap and easily accessible compound for crosslinking [89].

4. Collagen-based formulations for drug delivery

Traditional drugs have been the main concern to effectively treat the several diseases. The introduction of classical drug in therapeutics at high concentrations generally develops the substantial and sometimes severe consequences. The development of effective DDS for the efficacious augmentation of particular drug at desired target and at optimal concentrations for necessary duration has been the critical concern of clinical investigations and research since several years. To achieve the targeted or controlled local drug delivery, both synthetic and natural drug delivery materials are playing the important role.

At present, DDS have been developed based on polymers, nanomaterials and lipids etc. for the attachment or encapsulation of drugs to target the delivery or controlled release for long duration [90, 91]. Collagen based biomaterials or composite materials have become the important DDS due to specific pore size for active drug or principal load, effective fibrillar network, enzymatic degradation, long term stability *in vivo*, biocompatibility, low antigenicity, highly reduced toxicity and safety features [92]. The chemical modifications of –OH, $-NH_2$ and –COOH groups on collagen molecule making it more relevant and promising candidate in the domain of biomedicine. Collagen based biomaterials can be formulated into different forms according to desired medical application of drug delivery as mentioned in **Figure 3**. Various types of collagen based bioformulations such as hydrogels, films, sponges, scaffolds, matrices, aqueous injections, microspheres, micro-particles, micro-beads, NPs, nano-composites, nanofibres, shields, inserts, tubes, coatings, monolithic devices, implants and dressings etc. are applied for various drug delivery applications, tissue growth and regeneration. In **Table 2**, the type of formulations, synthetic or natural polymeric support material, active compound or drug and specific biomedical application has been summarized.

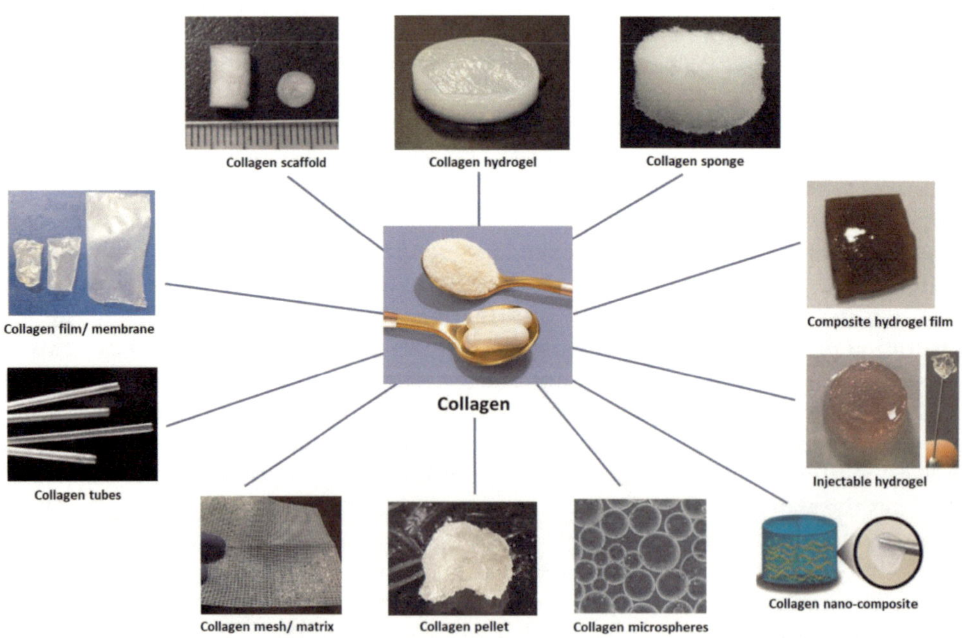

Figure 3.
Different types of collagen based biomaterials used for drug delivery.

Delivery form	Collagen/ collagen composite	Drug/active substance	Medicinal application	References
Gel/ hydrogel	Collagen	Keterolac	Inflammation	[93]
—	Collagen	TA	Drug release and kinetics	[94]
—	Collagen	NGF-β	Sustained delivery and corneal regeneration	[95]
—	Collagen	*Apis mellifera* royal jelly	Delivery vehicle for wound healing	[96]
—	Collagen	Curcumin	Controlled anti-proteolytic and pro-angiogenic efficacy	[97]
—	Gelatin	Essential oil of *Eupatorium adenophorum*	Antibacterial wound dressing	[98]
—	Collagen/ ALG	BSA	Ocular drug delivery	[46]
—	Collagen/ ALG	—	Cell proliferation	[48]
—	Collagen/ HEMA	GA, naproxen	Drug release, antimicrobial potential	[29]
—	Collagen/ Fe_3O_4 NPs	Fluorescein	Delivery, release and cell viability	[99]
—	Collagen/ CHS	QHREDGS	Myocardial infarction	[100]
—	Gelatin/ CHS/ ALG	5-FU	Anti cancer drug delivery	[49]
—	Collagen/ ALG	Methylene blue imiquimod	Combinatorial photothermal and immune tumor therapy	[101]
—	Collagen/ CHS	Tumor necrosis factor-α (TNF- α)	Drug delivery and tissue filler	[50]
—	Collagen/ graphene oxide (GO)	FGF-2	Controlled release	[102]
—	Collagen/ TA/ Poly-ethylenimine (PEI)	Doxorubicin (DOX)	Cancer therapy and antibacterial activity	[103]
—	Collagen/ CHS	—	Neuropathic diabetic foot ulcer (DBU) treatment	[104]
—	Collagen/ 1-ethyl-3-methylimidazolium acetate/ microbial transglutaminase	—	Controlled biodegradation	[86]
—	Collagen/ carrageenan	Allopurinol	Drug delivery and bioavailability	[105]
—	Collagen/ PLGA/ poly-lactic acid (PLA)/ poly-ε-caprolactone (PCL)	Spironolactone	Drug delivery	[106]
—	Collagen/ CHS	cell-penetrating peptide (CPP) (Oligoarginine, R8)	Wound healing and antimicrobial activity	[107]

Delivery form	Collagen/ collagen composite	Drug/active substance	Medicinal application	References
—	Collagen/ CHS	Thymosin β4(Tβ4)	Epicardial cell migration and angiogenesis	[108]
Hydrogel as aqueous injection	Collagen	Cisplatin, vinblastine, 5-FU, ^{111}In or ^{90}Y labeled monoclonal antibodies	Tumor treatment	[109–111]
—	Collagen	Transforming growth factor (TGF)-β, FGF, Insulin, growth hormone (GH)	Wound healing and repair	[112–114]
—	Collagen/ CMC	Interleukin (IL)-10	Retinal ischemia/ reperfusion therapy	[52]
—	Collagen/ CHS	Nanobodies: 2D5 and KPU	Tumor treatment in cancer therapy	[115]
—	Collagen/ ALG	Doxycycline	Vision-threatning diseases	[116]
Films	Collagen	Medroxyprogesterone acetate	Drug release	[117]
—	Collagen	Tetracycline, antibiotics	—	[118, 119]
—	Collagen	Platelet derived growth factor (PDGF)	Sustained release	[120]
—	Collagen	Proteins and polysaccharides	—	[121]
—	Collagen	Aloe vera	Enhanced biological avtivity	[32]
—	Collagen	Silver sulfadiazine	Antibacterial activity	[122]
—	Collagen	L-cysteine hydrochloride	Drug delivery	[123]
—	Collagen	—	Anti-aging activity	[124]
—	Collagen	Thymol	Antibacterial activity	[125]
—	Collagen/ elastin	—	Cell adhesion and viability	[126]
	Collagen/ PVA	Recombinant human growth hormone (rhGH)	Drug delivery	[127]
—	Collagen/ calcium phosphate	—	Cell adhesion, proliferation, differentiation, mineralization	[128]
—	Collagen/ polyurethane (PUR)	GF	Cell adhesion, proliferation and growth	[129]
—	Collagen/ carboxymethyl guar gum	Ceftazidime	Drug release, antibacterial activity	[130]
—	Collagen/ CHS	Gentamicin sulfate	Antibiotic release	[51]

Delivery form	Collagen/ collagen composite	Drug/active substance	Medicinal application	References
—	Collagen/ CHS	DOX	Cancer treatment	[131]
—	Collagen/ CHS	Lidocaine, tetracaine, benzocaine	Wound healing	[132]
—	Collagen/ CHS/ HA	Gentamicin sulfate	Antibiotic release	[133]
—	Collagen/ GO	Ovalbumin (OVA)	Sustained release	[134]
—	Collagen/ CHS	Allantoin and lidocaine	Wound healing	[135]
—	Collagen / CHS/ GO/ EDC	Basic fibroblast growth factor (bFGF)	Wound dressing	[136]
Membrane	Collagen/ PLGA	Vancomycin, gentamicin and lidocaine	Antibiotic activity	[137]
—	Collagen/ CHS	Nifedipine and propranolol hydrochloride	Cardiac disease	[138]
—	Collagen/ CHS	Nifedipine	Transdermal delivery	[139]
—	Collagen/ PVA	Ciprofloxacin hydrochloride	Antibacterial activity and treatment of ulcerative keratitis	[27]
Scaffold	Collagen as PURACOL®	Human antimicrobial peptide (AMP) cathelicidin LL37	Antimicrobial activity and cytotoxicity	[140]
—	Collagen	polyethylenimine (PEI)-plasmid DNA (pDNA) encoding PDGF-B complexes	Bone regeneration and gene delivery	[141]
—	Collagen/ CHS	Ibuprofen	Thermoresponsive scaffold	[142]
—	Collagen/ CHS	bFGF	Wound healing and skin tissue engineering	[143]
—	Collagen	N,N,N-trimethyl chitosan chloride (TMC)/ plasmid DNA encoding VEGF.	Angiogenesis and gene delivery vector	[144]
—	Collagen	BMP	Periodontal healing	[145]
—	Gelapin-Simvastatin Scaffolds	Simvastatin	Bone defect healing	[146]
—	Collagen/ CHS/ ALG	Curcumin	Diabetic wound healing	[147]
—	Collagen/ CHS	Norfloxacin	Skin regeneration	[148]
—	Collagen/ elastin	Penta-galloyl glucose (PGG)	Diabetes related complications	[149]
—	Collagen / HAP	PTHrP 107–111, pentapetide	Thermal drug release	[150]
—	Collagen/ CHS/ chondroitin (CHD)	PLGA microspheres	Tissue engineering	[151]

Delivery form	Collagen/ collagen composite	Drug/active substance	Medicinal application	References
—	Collagen/ PEI polyplexes	collagen-mimetic peptide (CMP)	Release kinetics and improved gene activity	[152]
—	Collagen/ CS	Platelet-rich plasma (PRP)	Growth factor release and wound healing	[153]
—	Collagen / HAP	BMP, alendronate	Bone regeneration	[154]
—	Collagen/ CHS	Curcumin nanoparticles	Wound healing and gene expression	[155]
Sponge	Collagen	Growth factors (GFs), FGF, BMPs	Wound healing and tissue regeneration	[156–159]
—	Collagen	Gentamicin, cefotaxim, fusidic acid, clindamycin	Wound healing	[160]
—	Collagen	All trans-retinoic acid	Cervical dysplasia	[161]
—	Collagen	Niflumic acid	Drug delivery and release	[162]
—	Collagen	Gentamicin	Wound infection	[163]
—	Collagen	BMP-2	Drug delivery comparison	[164]
—	Collagen/ PLGA	—	Cell attachment and cytotoxicity	[165]
—	Collagen/ CHS	Dexamethasone	Oral muscositis	[166]
—	Collagen/ PLGA	Gentamicin	Tissue regeneration	[167]
—	Collagen/ PCL/ HA	Methylene blue and curcumin	Sustained drug release kinetics	[168]
Matrix	Collagen	Ampicillin	Drug release	[169]
—	Collagen	Cisplatin	Local cancer therapy	[170]
—	Collagen/ PEI/ DNA complex	—	Tissue repair	[171]
—	Collgen as INFUSE® bone graft and MASTERGRAFT®	Recombinant bone morphogenetic protein-2 (rhBMP-2)	Bone fracture and spinal fusion	[172]
—	Collagen/ HA	—	Tissue development	[173]
—	Collagen/ chondroitin-6-sulphate (CS)	rhBMP-4	Drug delivery	[174]
—	Collagen/ heparin	—	Cofibrillogenesis	[175]
—	Collagen/ tri-calcium phosphate (CP)	Chondroinductive growth factor	Osteochondral tissue repair	[176]
3-D microsphere	Collagen	Glial derived neurotrophic factor (GDNF)	Controlled proliferation	[177]
—	Collagen	BMP-2	Local delivery	[178]

Delivery form	Collagen/ collagen composite	Drug/active substance	Medicinal application	References
—	Collagen/ CHS/ nano-HAP	—	Drug delivery	[179]
—	Collagen/ BC	BSA	Potential DDS	[54]
—	Collagen/ ALG	GDNF	Neurodegenerative diseases	[180]
—	Collagen/ BC	BMP-2	Adhesion, proliferation and osteogenic differentiation	[53]
—	Collagen/ ALG	BMP-4	Proliferation and differentiation	[181]
Microparticles	Collagen	Retinol, tretinoin, tetracain, lidocain	Drug delivery	[182]
—	Collagen	Cyclosporine	Allograft implantation	[183, 184]
—	Collagen	Glucocorticosteroids	Drug delivery	[185]
—	Collagen	Lysozyme	Protein delivery	[186]
—	Collagen/ hydroxyl ethylcellulose	Retinol	Drug delivery	[187]
—	Collagen/ poly oxyethylated sorbitan ester	Ethacridine lactate	Drug delivery	[188]
—	Collagen/ CHS/ CP	Glycolic acid	Tissue regeneration	[189]
Micro-beads	Collagen/ fibrin	Insulin like growth factor (IGF)-1	Regeneration of urethral sphincter muscle	[190]
Nanoparticle	Collagen	Estrogen (17-beta-estradiol-hemihydrate)	Delivery in hormone replacement therapy	[191]
—	Gelatin/ ALG/ Fe_3O_4	Doxorubicin hydrochloride	Cancer chemotherapy	[192]
—	Collagen/ CHS	Doxorubicin hydrochloride	Advanced cancer chemotherapy	[193]
—	Collagen peptide/ calcium/ ALG	—	Calcium supplementation	[194]
—	Collagen / Ferritin/ TaO NPs	TGF-β1	Sustained release, imaging and regeneration of oral tissue	[195]
—	Collagen/ ALG/ Ag	—	Wound healing	[47]
—	Atelocollagen	siRNA duplex	Delivery for gene silencing	[196]
Nanocomposite	Collagen/ bacterial cellulose (BC)/ apatite	Osteogenic growth peptide (OGP)	Bone regeneration	[197]
—	Collagen/ HAP/ ALG	Bone morphogenetic proteins (BMP)	Bone filler	[198]

Delivery form	Collagen/ collagen composite	Drug/active substance	Medicinal application	References
Nanofibres	Collagen/ PCL	—	Cell proliferation and migration	[199]
Inserts	Collagen	Gentamicin		[200]
—	Collagen	Erythromycin, erythromycin-estolate, penicillin-procaine	Infection, glaucoma	[201]
—	Collagen	Pilocarpine		[202]
Shields	Collagen	Tobramycin	Infection, mycosis	[203]
—	Collagen	Vancomycin	Infection, mycosis	[204]
—	Collagen	Gentamicin	Infection, mycosis	[205]
—	Collagen	Netilmycin	Infection, mycosis	[206]
—	Collagen	Amphotericin B	Glaucoma, inflammation	[207]
—	Collagen	Polymyxin B sulphate	Glaucoma, inflammation	[208]
—	Collagen	5-fluorouracil (5-FU)	Glaucoma, inflammation	[209]
—	Collagen	Steroids	Glaucoma, inflammation	[209, 210]
Monolithic devices	Collagen	Minocycline, lysozyme	Periodontitis	[211]
—	Collagen	Interleukin-2 (IL-2)	Drug delivery	[212]
—	Collagen	Interferon	Drug delivery	[213]
Tubes	Collagen/ silk fibroin	—	Vascular tissue engineering	[214]
Coating for composite	Collagen/ poly-L-lactic acid (PLLA)	—	Cell compatibility	[215]
—	Collagen as enteric coating	Gastro-resistant tablets	Delayed release	[216]
Implant	Collagen	Gentamicin	Prevention of surgical site infection	[217]
—	Collagen	PS1 as antineoplastic glycan	Antitumor activity	[218]
—	Collagen/ PCL	—	Corneal tissue regeneration	[219]
Dressing	Collagen/ ALG/ HA	Ampicillin	Wound healing and antimicrobial activity	[220]
—	Collagen/ CHS/ glucan	A. vera	Antibacterial activity, wound healing of chronic wounds and ulcers	[221]

Table 2.
Application of collagen and collagen based material in drug delivery systems (DDS).

4.1 Gel/hydrogel

Hydrogels are three dimensional (3-D) crosslinked arrangements of similar or different types of polymeric molecules with the property of absorbing and retaining the optimum quantity of water or biological fluid without degrading or losing the network structure. The material can be categorized as hydrogel, if the water content in the material is at least 10% of the total weight or volume of hydrogel [38]. The water molecules in the hydrogel provide the freedom of flexibility to design the natural tissue like environment. Hydrogels can be synthetic or natural with different chemical constituents and having different mechanical, physical and chemical attributes according to biomedical application. Hydrogels can be hydrophilic or hydrophobic in nature. Hydrophilic hydrogels possess hydroxyl (–OH), amine ($–NH_2$), carboxyl (–COOH), amide ($–CONH–CONH_2$) and sulphonic ($–SO_3H$) group for the swelling and absorbing property. The hydrophobic polymers show low swelling feature despite having improved mechanical, physical or chemical strength.

Drug transport within hydrogel can be regulated by altering the network/mesh size or the interactions with drugs using chemical methods [172, 222]. If the loaded drug is smaller than the crosslinked network of hydrogel, it can simply diffuse through the hydrogel while the larger drug molecules are entrapped within the hydrogel network and can be released after the degradation of the mesh. The biopolymer and its crosslinked network can be degenerated via slow hydrolysis of peptide or ester linkage or cleaving the thiol-related bonds, or through the enzymatic activity [223]. By the incorporation of non-covalent or covalent drug-matrix interactions, drug release from the hydrogel can be tuned [224, 225]. The characters mainly mesh size, crosslinking chemistry and drug interactions facilitate the better handling of drug transport through hydrogel. ECM-based hydrogels are the preferred choice for local drug delivery due to mechanical and biochemical support through cell-matrix interactions and diffusion and infiltration of small drug molecules in between crosslinked polymeric network [172].

Collagen alone is used for the delivery of several drugs and active principles such as keterolac, nerve growth factor (NGF)-β, TA, curcumin and royal jelly etc. for various biomedical purposes like anti-inflammation, corneal regeneration, drug release and kinetics, angiogenesis and wound healing, respectively. According to Ramírez et al. [96] type I collagen hydrogel extracellular vehicles (EVs) with *Apis mellifera* royal jelly displayed effective wound healing to stimulate mesenchymal stem cell (MSC) migration and inhibition of biofilm formation by *Staphylococcus aureus* along with stable release kinetics up to 7 days. Curcumin crosslinked collagen aerogel system expressed the enhanced physical and mechanical features and controlled anti-proteolytic and pro-angiogenic potential, made them appropriate 3D scaffolds for medicine purposes. Here, curcumin as a nutraceutical was used as a crosslinker for further usage [97]. In a study by Chuysinuan et al. [98], gelatin-based hydrogel was prepared by mixing gelatin with GTA crosslinker and essential oil of *Eupatorium adenophorum* and applied on patients with open wound to assess the wound healing and anti-bacterial properties by analyzing release profiles.

Collagen-based composite materials with synthetic (CMC, PVA, PCL, PEMA, HEMA, polyurethane (PUR) etc.) or natural (CL, bacterial cellulose (BC), CHS, ALG, HA, GAGs etc.) polymers have major roles in biomedicine. Liu et al. [46] developed a composite of collagen-ALG with suitable mechanical strength and optical clarity to support human corneal epithelial cell growth using bovine serum albumin (BSA) as a model drug. The hydrogel system could be applied as therapeutic lens in patients with corneal illnesses. Collagen-based hydrogel preparation by mixing of acrylamide and 2-hydroxy ethyl methacrylate (HEMA) was used as DDS for linear release profile of gallic acid (GA) and naproxen up to 36 hours for wound healing. Addition of metal NPs such as Ag and Cu in this collagen-HEMA hydrogel films showed antimicrobial potential against *Escherichia coli, Bacillus subtilis* and *S. aureus* [29]. Bettnini et al. [99] prepared the porous collagen-based hydrogel scaffold with iron oxide (Fe_3O_4) NPs for the release of fluorescein and biocompatibility, cell viability of 3 T3 fibroblasts cells and proposed the safety and applications in tissue engineering and drug delivery. Reis et al. [100] developed the collagen-CHS thermoresponsive hydrogel conjugated with angiopoietin-1 derived peptide glutamine-histidine-arginine-glutamic acid-aspartic acid-glycine-serine peptide (QHREDGS) for the survival and maturation of cardiomyocytes. Hydrogels with high peptide load showed better morphology, viability, metabolic activity, success rate of beating as compared to hydrogels with low peptide concentration and control groups.

Graphene oxide (GO) sheets were inserted into the collagen-based hydrogels for the controlled release of fibroblast growth factor (FGF)-2 to induce pluripotent stem cell culture. Low permeability of GO sheets allowed the release of FGF-2 in controlled and regulated fashion while the FGF-2 interacted with collagen through electrostatic forces and partial hydrogen bonding. The release profile of FGF-2 was attained up to 400 hours using three different concentrations of GO and showed the fabricated hydrogel for better release of growth factors (GFs) for biomedical application [102]. Choi et al. [103] developed the collagen-TA-poly ethylenimine (PEI) hydrogel with layer-by-layer self-assembled films to overcome the problem of poor mechanical strength and fast release of inserted drug. Doxorubicin (DOX) was used as model cancer therapy drug. The multifunctional hydrogels showed sustained and controlled release up to 6–7 days without any cytotoxic effects along with antibacterial property against Gram positive and negative bacteria and higher strength to compression load.

Injectable hydrogels are the promising materials for cancer treatment and controlled delivery. With the minimal invasive processes injectable hydrogels can be located and remained at required position and also mitigate the irregular shape defects after the implantation. Aqueous injections of hydrogels could be used in biomedicine field such as drug release, wound healing, repair, tumor treatment, tissue regeneration, ocular/retinal disorders and cancer therapy etc. Fan et al. [115] designed the hydrogel prepared from tilapia skin collagen and CHS for the delivery of model nanobodies- 2D5 and KPU. The hydrogel was biodegradable and expedited the release of nanobodies and could pave the way for tumor treatment. Carboxymethyl cellulose (CMC)-collagen based aqueous injectable hydrogel showed promising antioxidative and drug carrier benefits to treat the retinal ischaemia or reperfusion injury in rat models and could be applied for drug based treatment of retinal illnesses in humans. Animals were treated with interleukin (IL)-10 loaded hydrogels and expressed better therapeutic results of restoration of retinal structures and reduced retinal apoptosis, significantly decreased retinal oxidative stress in comparison to control group [52].

4.2 Films/membranes

The films or membranes are very thin and flexible layer of biopolymers with or without plasticizer having optical and mechanical anisotropy with very high tensile strength making them suitable for various medical applications of sustained drug release, cell adhesion, proliferation, differentiation, cancer treatment, wound healing and tissue regeneration. The thin films are the prominent material to target sensitive locations not possible with other formulations like liquid or tablets [226]. Thin films exhibited the improvised onset of drug activity, decreased dose quantity or frequency and augmented drug efficacy, reduced side effects by drug and extensive metabolism [227, 228].

Gil et al. [122] developed the innovative chromium free-collagen film for slow drug release carrier for skin burn related complications like ulcers and infected wounds. The biocompatible films were tested for drug silver sulfadiazine and its antibacterial potential against *Pseudomonas aeruginosa*, *E. coli*, *Micrococcus luteus*, *S. aureus*, *Proteus vulgaris* and *Klebsiella pneumoniae*. The findings proposed the effective strategy for Chromium (Cr) removal from leather waste and generation of environment friendly material could be transformed into collagen films, promising candidate for drug carriers. The use of biocompatible, recyclable, biodegradable natural materials has become tremendously increased in recent decades. Langasco et al. [123] developed the natural collagen films from marine sponges for topical drug delivery application. L-cysteine loaded films were analyzed for different drug concentrations and drying parameters. The films showed the healing potential of cysteine, acted as biocompatible carrier to absorb excess of wound exudate along with drug release. The films could be the promising material and might behave as bioactive, biomimetic drug carrier for effective wound healing. Jana et al. [130] synthesized the fish scale collagen-carboxymethyl guar gum film loaded with broad spectrum antibiotic ceftazidime. Around 90–95% of ceftazidime was released after 96 hours at physiological pH. *In vitro* study on NIH 3 T3 fibroblast cell line showed the biocompatibility of crosslinked film and antibacterial results exhibited the inhibition of *S. aureus* and *P. aeruginosa*.

Collagen-CHS based films/membranes are important biomaterials and used for antibiotic release, wound healing, cancer treatment, transdermal delivery, cardiac illness, tissue engineering. Martino et al. [132] formulated the collagen-CHS film for the delivery of mixture of local anesthetics compounds- lidocaine, tetracaine and benzocaine. The films were developed by rapid, cost effective and highly reproducible casting approach. The films showed good mechanical strength and flexibility with high water permeability. The anesthetics were uniformly distributed in the film and controlled released from 6 to 24 hours. The film exhibited *in vitro* non-cytotoxicity, cell proliferative and biocompatibility properties against human dermal fibroblast cells making it better candidate for drug release and proliferation. Liu et al. [136] fabricated the collagen-CHS-GO composite film using EDC as crosslinker loaded with basic FGF for effective wound healing through controlled release. The film had improved thermal endurance and higher degree of crosslinking for advanced mechanical strength due to GO. This novel DDS prevented the initial sudden release and loss of bioactive potential of basic FGF *in vivo* and *in vitro*. In cultured L929 fibroblasts, the film showed good biocompatibility in terms of cell adhesion and proliferation. These films were implanted on rats showed the wound remodeling to repair full thickness skin wound. So these films were promising substitute as wound dressing material for drug delivery with wound healing. Daja et al. [27] developed the collagen/PVA anionic membrane for drug carrier of ciprofloxacin hydrochloride along with antibacterial efficacy and its application in the treatment of ulcerative keratitis. The membrane provided the sustained DDS and inhibited the growth of *S. aureus* and *E. coli* during 48 hours. The membrane had proper mechanical strength, water amount, hydrophilicity, permeability and pH without any stress to cornea during interaction. The collagen fibrils in membrane decreased stromal damage and improved the epithelium regeneration. The formulated membranes were cost-effective and secured biomaterial for the treatment of corneal ulcers in patients.

4.3 Scaffolds/sponges/matrices

Scaffolds are collagen sponges or matrices with three dimensional network structures. Scaffolds can be obtained with various synthesis approaches of freeze drying, electrospinning and 3D printing etc. The freeze drying is the most effective method preserving the structure and native or inherent properties of collagen along with loaded drug/active principle in the scaffold. Collagen-based scaffolds or matrices are the important and favorable materials for bone, skin and tissue regeneration, angiogenesis, gene delivery, wound healing and repair, sustained drug release and improved gene expression. Now a days several commercially available collagen-based sponges in the market are Collarx®, Collatamp® G, Collatamp®EG Sulmycin® Implant, Garamycin® Schwamm, Duracol®, Duracoll®, Gentacol®, Gentacoll®, Garacol®, Garacoll® and Cronocol® - Gentamicin surgical implants.

Elangovan et al. [141] developed the non-viral gene delivery system for bone regeneration with the help of collagen scaffold to deliver the PEI-plasmid DNA encoding platelet derived growth factor (PDGF)-B complexes. The complexes expressed low cytotoxicity and markedly higher proliferation of human bone marrow stromal cells in contrast to scaffold without DNA and PDGF-B. In rats model the complexes exhibited higher bone volume followed the 4 weeks of grafting in comparison to empty scaffolds. The results advocated the use of non-viral scaffolds for bone regeneration along with gene delivery vehicle in clinical applications. Collagen-based biopolymers are one of the most important biomaterials to formulate the matrices in the field of tissue engineering due to significant non-toxicity, biocompatibility and resorptive potential. López-Noriega et al. [150] designed the collagen-hydroxyapatite (HAP) scaffold with covalently attached thermoresponsive liposomes. The encapsulated drug with pro-osteogenic and anti-osteoclastic properties was $PTHrP_{107-111}$, a pentapeptide. The regulated release of pentapeptide was correlated with enhanced expression of osteopontin and osteocalcin genes in cultured pre-osteoblastic MC3T3-E1 cells. This scaffold medicated drug release and cell regeneration has vast potential for various types of tissue regeneration.

Collagen-based 3D biomaterials are broadly used in the field of biomedicine for their properties of biocompatibility, inherent bioactivity to induce cell proliferation, hemostatic and low antigenicity. A porous and highly structured biomaterial such as sponges or matrices promotes the flexibility, permeability and biomimicry [229, 230]. Crosslinking or amalgamation of natural or synthetic biopolymers improvises the shortcomings of collagen polymer alone in terms of physico-chemical and biological parameters. Alagha et al. [166] prepared the porous muco-adhesive collagen-CHS biosponge as DDS for dexamethasone to treat the oral mucositis. The sponge was characterized by X-ray, FTIR, SEM, DSC and swelling behavior. The collagen-CHS sponge showed regulated drug release up to 10 hours as compared to collagen sponge for 5 hours. David et al. [168] fabricated the collagen-PCL-HA macroporous sponge to deliver the model drug methylene blue and curcumin. Several parameters such as absorption, water uptake, drug loading and delivery along with mechanical and structural features were examined for the developed sponge. In comparison to control group, the sponge showed sustained release kinetics for drugs and making the sponge as future material for applications of wound dressing and lab models.

Collagen matrices are able to deliver the gene or plasmid DNA in cultured cells and alter the gene expression in tissue engineering. Orsi et al. [171] formulated the bioactivated collagen-PEI-DNA complex to control the gene expression and attract the specific cell type. The transfected NIH3T3 cells with matrix-PEI-DNA complex secreted the plasmid encoded protein to promote the tissue repair and regeneration. The developed matrix could be the new approach for tissue repair.

4.4 3-D microspheres/ microparticles/micro-beads

Microspheres, microparticles or micro-beads are spherical particles with large surface to volume ratio for improved drug delivery, growth factors and broad surface area for cellular interactions to other biomolecules [28]. The size of collagen-based microparticles ranging from 3 to 40 μm. Berndt et al. [231] developed the collagen microspheres encapsulated astrocytes crosslinked with poly (ethylene glycol) tetrasuccinimidyl glutarate (4S-StarPEG) as growth enhancing and carrier for injured spinal cord. Astrocytes were transfected with plasmids encoding nerve growth factor (NGF)-ires-enhanced green fluorescent protein (EGFP) genes and then added to the culture of rat dorsal root ganglion and significantly improved growth was observed. The report showed the potential of microspheres as carrier of astrocytes for neural tissue regeneration. Zhang et al. [53] formulated the 3-D microsphere of collagen-BC-bone morphogenic protein (BMP)-2 for bone tissue augmentation. The 3D microporous microspheres effectively enhanced the adhesion, proliferation and osteogenic differentiation of mice MC3T3-E1 cells and expressed adequate biocompatibility.

Marine based collagen from jellyfish species *Catostylus tagi* was used to develop the microparticles formulation for sustained delivery of lysozyme and α-lactalbumin. The collagen microparticles were crosslinked with EDC and investigation of lysozyme activity was retained throughout the crosslinking and encapsulation process. These microparticles from marine collagen could be the promising material for controlled release of therapeutic proteins [186]. Yang and Fang [232] developed the microporous nano-HAP/collagen/phosphatidylserine scaffolds embedding collagen microparticles for the sustained release of steroidal saponins for bone tissue engineering in cultured MC-3 T3-E1 cells. The scaffolds provided scope for spatial and temporally controlled drug delivery and deposition at wounded site and reduction in adverse side effects. Vardar et al. [190] formulated the novel injectable collagen-fibrin microfluidic system loaded with recombinant insulin like growth factor-1 (α_2PI_{1-8}-MMp-IGF-1) to treat the urinary incontinence. The natural crosslinker genipin was used for collagen modification. The microbeads showed slow release of GF and positive cell behavior for the induction of *in vivo* smooth muscle regeneration for effective management of urinary incontinence.

4.5 Nanoparticles/ nanocomposites/nanofibres

Nanomaterials within the size of 1–100 nm are one of the best materials with admirable biochemical and pharmacological attributes [233]. Biological protein-based NPs are applied in different applications due to eco-friendly nature and biocompatibility and replacing the synthetic materials. Collagen is the preferred NP substance and by direct or indirect crosslinking to collagen NPs provide better substitute for protein based drug delivery vehicle [234]. The crosslinking of collagen with NPs is the new strategy to enhance the mechanical and physical strength of collagen tissue for various applications. Metal oxide NPs such as iron oxide (Fe_3O_4), zinc oxide (ZnO), alumina oxide (Al_2O_3), tantalum oxide (TaO), Al_2O_3-ZrO_2 and Fe_3O_4-ZnO improve the mechanical features of collagen-based biomaterials [99, 195, 235]. The metallic NPs provided broad spectrum antimicrobial, antioxidative and anti-inflammatory attributes [236, 237] to collagen based material and serve as an alternative to toxic chemical crosslinkers and impede the collagen degradation by physical crosslinking. These features advertise the use of NPs based collagen biopolymers in medical field such as targeted controlled drug delivery, cell targeting and tissue engineering. Choi et al. [195] prepared the collagen hydrogel containing the ferritin NPs, TaO NPs along with transforming growth factor (TGF)-β1 for the controlled release and imaging medium for regeneration of oral tissues.

NPs based biopolymers for cancer therapeutics are effectively utilized in recent years due to targeted and controlled release kinetics. Anandhakumar et al. [193] fabricated the collagen peptide-CHS NPs for encapsulation of standard cancer drug DOX in cancer therapy. The NPs showed high encapsulation capacity of DOX and pH regulated release. NPs with DOX expressed significant anti-proliferative activity against HeLa cells in contrast to normal cells. The NPs showed excellent biocompatibility with high power as smart DDS for cancer therapeutics. Zhang et al. [47] designed the collagen-ALG biocomposite doped with silver NPs (AgNPs) with antibacterial potential and applicable as wound dressing. The biocomposite exhibited insignificant *in vitro* toxicity at lower concentrations of AgNPs and also inhibited the growth of *S. aureus* and *E. coli*. Saska et al. [197] fabricated the nanocomposite of BC-collagen-apatite and osteogenic growth peptide (OGP) for bone tissue regeneration. The OGP containing nanocomposite triggered the early development of osteoblastic phenotype and elevated cellular growth without any cytotoxic, genotoxic or mutagenic adverse effects. The nanocomposite could be the promising future biomaterial for bone tissue engineering.

4.6 Inserts/shields/monolithic devices or pellets

The approach of applying ocular collagen inserts to administer the drug for prolonged period was started in early 1970s. The inserts were films or as molded rods or wafers of collagen incorporated with drug such as pilocarpine, penicillin-procaine, erythromycin, erythromycin esolate and gentamicin etc. in the form of eyedrops, ointments and subconjunctival injections to treat the cornea related disorders [200–202]. In the late 1980s researches on inserts were overtaken by shields which became commercially available in the market in reproducible manner [7].

Collagen shields were formulated as corneal bandages/dressings to facilitate the wound healing, allow sufficient oxygen transmission, lubricate the eye surface to minimize stress and to regenerate the corneal epithelial linings after corneal injury or damage, transplantation, radial keratomy, glaucoma, keratitis or cornea related disorders [238, 239]. These shields could be used as carrier to deliver the ophthalmic medication such as water soluble antibiotics- gentamicin, vancomycin, tobramycin, netilmicin, polymyxin B sulphate, trimethoprim, amphotericin B, pilocarpine and flurbiprofene sodium etc. [7]. The drug delivery aspect of shields is limited by transparency, reduced visual acuity, slight irritation, complex administration procedure and prolonged durability. In current scenario, the commercial formulations like Biocora®, ProshieldO®, MediLenso®, Irvine® and Chiron® etc. are showing better future for delivery of corticosteroids and subconjuctival antibiotics etc. [240].

Collagen minipellets are cylindrical injectable controlled release drug delivery vehicle. In 1992, Takeuchi [211] prepared the little rods of 1 mm in diameter and length of 15 mm of injectable collagen minipellet for the local delivery of minocycline and lysozyme to treat periodontitis. Fujioka et al. [241] used the injectable collagen minipellet to deliver interleukin (IL)-2 molecule. Maeda et al. [242] used the collagen minipellet as a carrier to deliver the recombinant human bone morphogenic protein (rhBMP)-2 to induce the bone formation in mice models. Lofthouse et al. [243] developed the degradable collagen minipellet infused with avidin and IL-1β as vaccine carrier for clostridial antigen into sheep and mice. Higaki et al. [244] fabricated the biodegradable collagen minipellet to deliver the tetanus and diphtheria toxoid as single dose vaccine delivery system in mice.

5. Conclusion

Protein-based biomaterials have excellent biocompatibility with minimal cytotoxicity and biodegradability and theirs physical, chemical and biological parameters can be altered according to biomedical application. Collagen, a major protein in animal body is the attractive biopolymers for the delivery of therapeutic drugs, growth factors, hormones, proteins/enzymes, gene and imaging probes in the field of drug delivery systems, wound healing, bone grafts, implants, tissue regeneration, ocular diseases, cosmetic surgery, reconstructive surgery and cardiac treatments.

The researchers are consistently designing the protein-based hybrid materials with desired physical, mechanical, chemical and biological properties. Collagen-based hybrid biomaterials can be formed with natural polymers like CHS, CL, ALG, gelatin, HA, CHD, HAP or the chemically modified form of these natural polymers or with synthetic polymer such as CMC, PVA, PCL, PEMA, PLA and PLGA etc. through various physical, chemical and enzymatic crosslinking approaches. Collagen-based biomaterials can be fabricated into variety of physical forms hydrogel, films or membranes, scaffolds or sponges, matrices, 3-D microspheres, microparticles, nanoparticles, nanocomposites, inserts, shields and pellets for drug based delivery of synthetic and natural active biocomponents in various fields of medical science. Collagen-based biomaterials have attracted the researchers to develop efficient and controlled therapeutic vehicles for clinical applications ensuring the patient compliance. The more efforts are needed to translate the clinical results into production scale with collaboration of researchers, material scientists, clinical doctors and industry.

Author details

Amit Kumar Verma
Department of Biosciences, Jamia Millia Islamia, Srinivasa Ramanujan Block, New Delhi, India

*Address all correspondence to: averma@jmi.ac.in

References

[1] Ahmed M, Verma AK, Patel R. Collagen extraction and recent biological activities of collagen peptides derived from sea-food waste: A review. Sustainable Chemistry and Pharmacy. 2020;**18**:100315. DOI: 10.1016/j.scp.2020.100315

[2] Zhang Y, Sun T, Jiang C. Biomacromolecules as carriers in drug delivery and tissue engineering. Acta Pharmaceutica Sinica B. 2018;**8**(1): 34-50. DOI: 10.1016/j.apsb.2017.11.005

[3] Jao D, Xue Y, Medina J, Hu X. Protein-based drug-delivery materials. Materials (Basel). 2017;**10**(5):517. DOI: 10.3390/ma100505517

[4] Zhang X, Zhang J, Shi. Mesoporousbioglass/silk fibroin scaffolds as a drug delivery system: Fabrication, drug loading and release *in vitro* and repair calvarial defects *in vivo*. Journal of Wuhan University of Technology-Materials Science Edition. 2014;**29**:401-406. DOI: 10.1007%2Fs11595-014-0929-0

[5] Albu MG, Titorencu I, Ghica MV. Collagen-based drug delivery systems for tissue engineering. In: Pignatello R, editor. Biomaterials Applications for Nanomedicine. London: InTech; 2011. pp. 333-358. Available from: http://www.intechopen.com/books/biomaterialsapplications-for-anomedicine/collagen-based-drug-delivery-systems-for-tissue-engineering

[6] Fujioka K, Maeda M, Hojo T, Sano A. Protein release from collagen matrices. Advanced Drug Delivery Reviews. 1998; **31**:247-266

[7] Friess W. Collagen – biomaterial for drug delivery. European Journal of Pharmaceutics and Biopharmaceutics. 1998;**45**:113-136

[8] Piez KA. Collagen. In: Encyclopaedia of Polymer Science and Engineering. New York: Wiley; 1985. pp. 699-727

[9] Bhagwat PK, Dandge PB. Collagen and collagenolytic proteases: A review. Biocatalysis and Agriculatral Biotechnology. 2018;**15**:43-55. DOI: 10.1016/j.bcab.2018.05.005

[10] Yang YJ, Jung D, Yang B, Hwang BH, Cha HJ. Aquatic proteins with repetitive motifs provide insights to bioengineering of novel biomaterials. Biotechnology Journal. 2014;**9**(12): 1493-1502. DOI: 10.1002/biot.201400070

[11] Addad S, Exposito J-Y, Faye C, Ricard-Blum S, Lethias C. Isolation, characterization and biological evaluation of jellyfish collagen for use in biomedical applications. Marine Drugs. 2011;**9**(6):967-983. DOI: 10.3390/md9060967

[12] Ricard-Blum S. The collagen family. In: Hynes R, Yamada K, editors. Additional Perspectives on Extracellular Matrix Biology. Cold Spring Harbor Perspectives in Biology. Cold Spring Harbor, New York: Cold Spring Harbor Laboratory Press; 2011. pp. 1-20. DOI: 10.1101/cshperspect.a004978

[13] Varanko A, Saha S, Chilkoti A. Recent trends in protein and peptide-based biomaterials for advanced drug delivery. Advanced Drug Delivery Reviews. 2020;**156**:133-187. DOI: 10.1016/j.addr.2020.08.008

[14] Gelse K, Pöschl E, Aigner T. Collagens - Structure, function, and biosynthesis. Advanced Drug Delivery Reviews. 2003;**55**:1531-1546. DOI: 10.1016/j.addr.2003.08.002

[15] Felician FF, Xia C, Qi W, Xu H. Collagen from marine biological sources

and medical applications. Chemistry & Biodiversity. 2018;**15**(5):e1700557. DOI: 10.1002/cbdv.201700557

[16] Wang D-A, Williams CG, Yang F, Elisseeff H. Enhancing the tissue-biomaterial interface: Tissue-initiated integration of biomaterials. Advanced Functional Materials. 2004;**14**(12): 1152-1159

[17] Hench LL, Ethridge EC. Biomaterials: An Interfacial Approach. New York: Academic Press; 1982. p. 385

[18] Raghavendra GM, Varaprasad K, Jayaramudu T. Biomaterials: Design, development and biomedical applications. In: Thomas S, Grohens Y, Ninan N, editors. Nanotechnology Applications for Tissue Engineering. Amsterdam: Elsevier Inc; 2015. DOI: 10.1016/B978-0-323-32889-0.00002-9

[19] Bronzino JD. The Biomedical Engineering Handbook. 2nd ed. Vol. 2. New York: CRC Press; 1999. p. 2896

[20] Helmus MN, Gibbons DF, Cebon D. Biocompatibility: Meeting a key functional requirement of next-generation medical devices. Toxicologic Pathology. 2008;**36**(1):70-80

[21] Yoruç BH, Şener BC. Biomaterials. In: Kara S, editor. A Roadmap of Biomedical Engineers and Milestones. Rijeka: InTech; 2012. Available from: http://www.intechopen.com/books/a-roadmap-of-biomedical-engineers-and-milestones/biomaterials

[22] Williams DF. Tissue biomaterial interactions. Journal of Materials Science. 1987;**22**(10):3421-3445. DOI: 10.1007/BF01161439

[23] Cheng W, Yan-hua R, Fang-gang N, Guo-anZ. The content and ratio of type I and III collagen in skin differ with age and injury. African Journal of Biotechnology. 2011;**10**:2524-2529

[24] Ramshaw JA, Peng YY, Glattauer V, Werkmeister J. Collagens as biomaterials. Journal of Materials Science: Materials in Medicine. 2009;**20**: 3-8. DOI: 10.1007%2Fs10856-008-3415-4

[25] Lin K, Zhang D, Macedo MH, Cui W, Sarmento B, Shen G. Advanced collagen-based biomaterials for regenerative biomedicine. Advanced Functional Materials. 2019;**29**:1804943. DOI: 10.1002/adfm.201804943

[26] Bretaud S, Guillon E, Karppinen S-M, Pihlajaniemi T, Ruggiero F. Collagen XV, a multifaceted multiplexin present across tissues and species. Matrix Biology Plus. 2020;**6-7**:100023. DOI: 10.1016/j.mbplus.2020.100023

[27] Daza JHU, Righetto GM, Chaud MV, Martins VCA, Camargo ILBC, Plepis AMG. PVA/anionic collagen membranes as drug carriers of ciprofloxacin hydrochloride with sustained antibacterial activity and potential use in the treatment of ulcerative keratitis. Journal of Biomaterials Applications. 2020;**35**(3):301-312. DOI: 10.1177/0885328220931733

[28] Geanaliu-Nicolae R-E, Andronescu E. Blended natural support materials-collagen based hydrogels used in biomedicine. Materials. 2020;**13**(24): 5641. DOI: 10.3390/ma13245641

[29] Sahiner M, Alpaslan D, Bitlisli BO. Collagen-based hydrogel films as drug-delivery devices with antimicrobial properties. Polymer Bulletin. 2014;**71**: 3017-3033. DOI: 10.1007/s00289-014-1235-x

[30] Parenteau-Bareil R, Gauvin R, Berthod F. Collagen-based biomaterials

for tissue engineering applications. Materials. 2010;**3**:1863-1887

[31] Antoine EE, Vlachos PP, Rylander MN. Review of collagen I hydrogels for bioengineered tissue microenvironments: Characterization of mechanics, structure, and transport. Tissue Engineering Part B Reviews. 2014;**20**(20):683-696. DOI: 10.1089/ten.TEB.2014.0086

[32] Andonegi M, Heras KL, Santos-Vizcaino E, Igartua M, Hernandez RM, Caba KDL, et al. Structure-properties relationship of chitosan/collagen films with potential for biomedical applications. Carbohydrate Polymers. 2020;**237**:116159. DOI: 10.1016/j.carbpol.2020.116159

[33] Rafat M, Li F, Fagerholm P, Lagali NS, Watsky MA, Munger R, et al. Peg-stabilized carbodiimide crosslinked collagen–chitosan hydrogels for corneal tissue engineering. Biomaterials. 2008; **29**:3960-3972. DOI: 10.1016/j.biomaterials.2008.06.017

[34] Broguiere N, Formica FA, Barreto G, Zenobi-Wong M. Sortase a as a cross-linking enzyme in tissue engineering. Acta Biomaterialia. 2018;**77**:182-190. DOI: 10.1016/j.actbio.2018.07.020

[35] Hamedi H, Moradi S, Hudson SM, Tonelli AE. Chitosan based hydrogels and their applications for drug delivery in wound dressings: A review. Carbohydrate Polymers. 2018;**1**(199): 445-460. DOI: 10.1016/j.carbpol.2018.06.114

[36] Wu X, Liu A, Wang W, Ye R. Improved mechanical properties and thermal-stability of collagen fiber based film by crosslinking with casein, keratin or SPI: Effect of crosslinking process and concentrations of proteins. International Journal of Biological Macromolecules. 2018;**109**:1319-1328. DOI: 10.1016/j.ijbiomac.2017.11.144

[37] Picheth GF, Pirich CL, Sierakowski MR, Woehl MA, Sakakibara CN, De Souza CF, et al. Bacterial cellulose in biomedical applications: A review. International Journal of Biological Macromolecules. 2017;**104**:97-106. DOI: 10.1016/j.ijbiomac.2017.05.171

[38] Bahram M, Mohseni N, Moghtader M. An introduction to hydrogels and some recent applications. In: Majee SB, editor. Emerging Concepts in Analysis and Applications of Hydrogels. Rijeka: IntechOpen; 2016. DOI: 10.5772/64301. Available from: https://www.intechopen.com/chapters/51535

[39] Voicu G, Geanaliu-Nicolae RE, Pîrvan A-A, Andronescu E, Florin I. Synthesis, characterization and bioevaluation of drug-collagen hybrid materials for biomedical applications. International Journal of Pharmaceutics. 2016;**510**:474-484. DOI: 10.1016/j.ijpharm.2015.11.054

[40] Ahmadi F, Oveisi Z, Samani SM, Amoozgar Z. Chitosan based hydrogels: Characteristics and pharmaceutical applications. Research in Pharmaceutical Sciences. 2015;**10**(1):1-16

[41] Voicu G, Geanaliu-Nicolae RE, Ghitulica CD, Ficai A, Grumezescu AM, Bleotu C. Synthesis, characterization and bioevaluation of irinotecan-collagen hybrid materials for biomedical applications as drug delivery systems in tumoral treatments. Central European Journal of Chemistry. 2013;**11**:2134-2143. DOI: 10.2478/s11532-013-0341-1

[42] Gu L, Shan T, Ma Y-X, Tay FR, Niu L-N. Novel biomedical applications of crosslinked collagen. Trends in Biotechnology. 2019;**37**:464-491. DOI: 10.1016/j.tibtech.2018.10.007

[43] Bazrafshan Z, Stylios GK. Spinnability of collagen as a biomimetic material: A review. International Journal of Biological Macromolecules. 2019; **15**(129):693-705. DOI: 10.1016/j.ijbiomac.2019.02.024

[44] Ardelean IL, Gudovan D, Ficai D, Ficai A, Andronescu E, Albu-Kaya MG, et al. Collagen/hydroxyapatite bone grafts manufactured by homogeneous/heterogeneous 3D printing. Materials Letters. 2018;**231**:179-182. DOI: 10.1016/j.matlet.2018.08.042

[45] Lee KY, Mooney DJ. Alginate: Properties and biomedical applications. Progress in Polymer Science. 2012;**37**(1): 106-126. DOI: 10.1016/j.progpolymsci.2011.06.003

[46] Liu W, Griffith M, Li F. Alginate microsphere-collagen composite hydrogel for ocular drug delivery and implantation. Journal of Materials Science: Materials in Medicine. 2008;**19**: 3365-3371. DOI: 10.1007/s10856-008-3486-2

[47] Zhang H, Peng M, Cheng T, Zhao P, Qiu L, Zhou J, et al. Silver nanoparticles-doped collagen–alginate antimicrobial biocomposite as potential wound dressing. Journal of Materials Science. 2018;**53**:14944-14952

[48] Sang L, Luo D, Xu S, Wang X, Li X. Fabrication and evaluation of biomimetic scaffolds by using collagen–alginate fibrillar gels for potential tissue engineering applications. Materials Science and Engineering: C. 2011;**31**(2): 262-271

[49] Chen X, Fan M, Tan H, Ren B, Yuan G, Jia Y, et al. Magnetic and self-healing chitosan-alginate hydrogel encapsulated gelatin microspheres via covalent cross-linking for drug delivery. Materials Science & Engineering: C. 2019;**101**:619-629. DOI: 10.1016/j.msec.2019.04.012

[50] Wang W, Itoh S, Aizawa T, Okawa A, Sakai K, Ohkuma T, et al. Development of an injectable chitosan/marine collagen composite gel. Biomedical Materials. 2010;**5**:065009. DOI: 10.1088/1748-6041/5/6/065009

[51] Sionkowska A, Kaczmarek B, Gadzała-Kopciuch R. Gentamicin release from chitosan and collagen composites. Journal of Drug Delivery Science and Technology. 2016;**35**:353-359. DOI: 10.1016/j.jddst.2016.09.001

[52] Mu H, Wang Y, Wei H, Lu H, Feng Z, Yu H, et al. Collagen peptide modified carboxymethyl cellulose as both antioxidant drug and carrier for drug delivery against retinal ischaemia/reperfusion injury. Journal of Cellular & Molecular Medicine. 2018;**22**:5008-5019. DOI: 10.1111/jcmm.13768

[53] Zhang W, Wang X-C, Li X-Y, Zhang L-L, Jiang F. A 3D porous microsphere with multistage structure and component based on bacterial cellulose and collagen for bone tissue engineering. Carbohydrate Polymers. 2020;**236**:116043. DOI: 10.1016/j.carbpol.2020.116043

[54] Zhang W, Wang X-C, Wang J-J, Zhang L-L. Drugs adsorption and release behavior of collagen/bacterial cellulose porous microspheres. International Journal of Biological Macromolecules. 2019;**140**:196-205. DOI: 10.1016/j.ijbiomac.2019.08.139

[55] Gorgieva S, Kokol V. Collagen- vs. gelatine-based biomaterials and their biocompatibility: Review and perspectives. In: Pignatello R, editor. Biomaterials Applications for Nanomedicine. Rijeka: IntechOpen;

2011. DOI: 10.5772/24118. Available from: https://www.intechopen.com/chapters/23617

[56] Tefft S, Bentz H, Estridge TD. Collagen and heparin matrices for growth factor delivery. Journal of Controlled Release. 1997;**48**(1):29-33

[57] Jaikumar D, Baskaran B, Vaidyanathan VG. Effect of chromium (III) gallate complex on stabilization of collagen. International Journal of Biological Macromolecules. 2017;**96**: 429-435. DOI: 10.1016/j.ijbiomac.2016.12.049

[58] Chen Y-C, Chen M, Gaffney EA, Borwn CP. Effect of crosslinking in cartilage-like collagen microstructures. Journal of Mechanical Behavior of Biomedical Materials. 2017;**66**:138-143. DOI: 10.1016/j.jmbbm.2016.10.006

[59] Kishore V, Iyer R, Frandsen A, Nguyen T-U. In vitro characterization of electrochemically compacted collagen matrices for corneal applications. Biomedical Materials. 2016;**11**:055008. DOI: 10.1088/1748-6041/11/5/055008

[60] Dias J, Diakonis VF, Lorenzo M, Gonzalez F, Porras K, Douglas S, et al. Corneal stromal elasticity and viscoelasticity assessed by atomic force microscopy after different cross linking protocols. Experimental Eye Research. 2015;**138**:1-5. DOI: 10.1016/j.exer.2015.06.015

[61] Aldahlawi NH, Hayes S, O'Brart DPS, Akhbanbetova A, Littlechild SL, Meek KM. Enzymatic resistance of corneas crosslinked using riboflavin in conjunction with low energy, high energy, and pulsed UVA irradiation modes. Investigative Ophthalmology & Visual Science. 2016;**57**:1547-1552. DOI: 10.1167/iovs.15-18769

[62] Martinez AW, Caves JM, Ravi S, Li W, Chaikof EL. Effects of crosslinking on the mechanical properties, drug release and cytocompatibility of protein polymers. Acta Biomaterialia. 2014;**10**: 26-33. DOI: 10.1016/j.actbio.2013.08.029

[63] van Luyn MJA, van Wachem PB, Damink LO, Dijkstra PJ, Feijen J, Nieuwenhuis P. Secondary cytotoxicity of crosslinked dermal sheep collagens during repeated exposure to human fibroblasts. Biomaterials. 1992;**13**: 1017-1024

[64] Charulatha V, Rajaram A. Dimethyl 3,3′-dithiobispropionimidate: A novel crosslinking reagent for collagen. Journal of Biomedical Materials Research. 2001;**54**:122-128

[65] Tang Z, Yue Y. Crosslinkage of collagen by polyglycidyl ethers. American Society for Artificial Internal Organs Journal. 1995;**41**:72-78

[66] Nishi C, Nakajima N, Ikada Y. In vitro evaluation of cytotoxicity of diepoxy compounds used for biomaterial modification. Journal of Biomedical Materials Research. 1995;**29**:829-834

[67] van Wachem PB, van Luyn MJA, Nieuwenhuis P, Koerten HK, Damink LO, Hoopen HT, et al. In vivo degradation of processed dermal sheep collagen evaluation with transmission electron microscopy. Biomaterials. 1991;**12**:215-223

[68] Pieper JS, Oosterhof A, Dijkstra PJ, Veerkamp JH, van Kuppevelt TH. Preparation and characterization of porous crosslinked collagenous matrixes containing bioavailable chondroitin sulfate. Biomaterials. 1999;**20**:847-858

[69] Nagaoka H, Nagaoka H, Walter R, Boushell LW, Miguez PA, Burton A, et al. Characterization of

genipin-modified dentin collagen. BioMed Research International. 2014: 702821. DOI: 10.1155/2014/702821

[70] Balakrishnan B, Jayakrishnan A. Self-cross-linking biopolymers as injectable in situ forming biodegradable scaffolds. Biomaterials. 2005;**26**(18): 3941-3951

[71] Mu C, Liu F, Cheng Q, Li H, Wu B, Zhang G, et al. Collagen cryogel cross-linked by dialdehyde starch. Macromolecular Materials and Engineering. 2010;**295**(2):100-107

[72] Sisson K, Zhang C, Farach-Carson MC, Chase DB, Rabolt JF. Evaluation of cross-linking methods for electrospun gelatin on cell growth and viability. Biomacromolecules. 2009;**10**(7):1675-1680

[73] Tan H, Wu B, Li C, Mu C, Li H, Lin W. Collagen cryogel cross-linked by naturally derived dialdehyde carboxymethyl cellulose. Carbohydrate Polymers. 2015;**129**:17-24. DOI: 10.1016/j.carbpol.2015.04.029

[74] Zhang X, Do MD, Casey P, Sulistio A, Qiao GG, Lundin L, et al. Chemical crosslinking of gelatin with natural phenolic compounds as studied by high-resolution NMR spectroscopy. Biomacromolecules. 2010;**11**(4): 1125-1132

[75] Kim S, Nimni ME, Yang Z, Han B. Chitosan/gelatin-based films crosslinked by proanthocyanidin. Journal of Biomedical Materials Research Part B: Applied Biomaterials. 2005;**75**(2): 442-450

[76] He L, Mu C, Ski J, Zhang Q, Shi B, Lin Q. Modification of collagen with a natural cross-linker, procyanidin. International Journal of Biological Macromolecules. 2011;**48**(2):354-359

[77] Jackson JK, Zhao J, Wong W, Burt HB. The inhibition of collagenase induced degradation of collagen by the galloyl-containing polyphenols tannic acid, epigallocatechin gallate and epicatechin gallate. Journal of Materials Science: Materials for Medicine. 2010;**2**: 1435-1443

[78] Pena C, Caba K, Eceiza A, Ruseckaite R, Mondragon I. Enhancing water repellence and mechanical properties of gelatin films by tannin addition. Bio/Technology. 2010;**101**:6836-6842

[79] Davidenko N, Bax DV, Schuster CF, Farndale RW, Hamaia SW, Best SM, et al. Optimisation of UV irradiation as a binding site conserving method for crosslinking collagen-based scaffolds. Journal of Materials Science: Materials in Medicine. 2016;**27**:14. DOI: 10.1007/s10856-015-5627-8

[80] Rowland CR, Colucci LA, Guilak F. Fabrication of anatomically-shaped cartilage constructs using decellularized cartilage-derived matrix scaffolds. Biomaterials. 2016;**91**:57-72. DOI: 10.1016/j.biomaterials.2016.03.012

[81] Krishnakumar GS, Gostynska N, Dapporto M, Campodoni E, Montesi M, Panseri S, et al. Evaluation of different cross-linking agents on hybrid biomimetic collagen-hydroxyapatite composites for regenerative medicine. International Journal of Biological Macromolecules. 2018;**106**:739-748. DOI: 10.1016/j.ijbiomac.2017.08.076

[82] Heck T, Faccio G, Richter M, Linda T-ML. Enzyme-catalyzed protein crosslinking. Applied Microbiology & Biotechnology. 2013;**97**:461-475. DOI: 10.1007/s00253-012-4569-z

[83] Jus S, Stachel I, Schloegl W, Pretzler M, Friess W, Meyer M, et al. Cross-linking of collagen with laccases and

tyrosinases. Materials Science and Engineering C. 2011;**31**(5): 1068-1077

[84] Wu X, Liu Y, Liu A, Wang W. Improved thermal-stability and mechanical properties of type I collagen by crosslinking with casein, keratin and soy protein isolate using transglutaminase. International Journal of Biological Macromolecules. 2017;**98**: 292-301. DOI: 10.1016/j.ijbiomac. 2017.01.127

[85] Zhao L, Li X, Zhao J, Ma S, Fan D, Zhu C, et al. A novel smart injectable hydrogel prepared by microbial transglutaminase and human-like collagen: Its characterization and biocompatibility. Materials *Science & Engineering. C*, Materials for Biological Applications. 2016;**68**:317-326. DOI: 10.1016/j.msec.2016.05.108

[86] Li X, Fan D. Smart collagen hydrogels based on 1-ethyl-3-methylimidazolium acetate and microbial transglutaminase for potential applications in tissue engineering and cancer therapy. ACS Biomaterials Science & Engineering. 2019;**5**(7):3523-3536. DOI: 10.1021/ acsbiomaterials.9b00393

[87] Makris EA, Responte DJ, Paschos NK, Hu JC, Athanasiou KA. Developing functional musculoskeletal tissues through hypoxia and lysyl oxidase-induced collagen cross-linking. Proceedings of National Academy of Sciences, USA. 2014;**111**(45):E4832-E4841. DOI: 10.1073/pnas.1414271111

[88] Choi Y, Kim HJ, Min KS. Effects of proanthocyanidin, a crosslinking agent, on physical and biological properties of collagen hydrogel scaffold. Restorative Dentistry Endodontics. 2016;**41**(4): 296-303. DOI: 10.5395/rde.2016.41. 4.296

[89] Oryan A, Kamali A, Moshiri A, Baharvand H, Daemi H. Chemical crosslinking of biopolymeric scaffolds: Current knowledge and future directions of crosslinked engineered bone scaffolds. International Journal of Biological Macromolecules. 2018;**107**:678-688. DOI: 10.1016/j.ijbiomac.2017.08.184

[90] Kanamala M, Wilson WR, Yang M, Palmer BD, Wu Z. Mechanisms and biomaterials in pH-responsive tumour targeted drug delivery: A review. Biomaterials. 2016;**85**:152-167. DOI: 10.1016/j.biomaterials.2016.01.061

[91] Liu D, Yang F, Xiong F, Gu N. The smart drug delivery system and its clinical potential. Theranostics. 2016;**6**: 1306-1323. DOI: 10.7150/thno.14858

[92] Andersen JT, Dalhus B, Viuff D, Ravn BT, Gunnarsen KS, Plumridge A, et al. Extending serum half-life of albumin by engineering neonatal c receptor (FcRn) binding. Journal of Biological Chemistry. 2014;**289**:13492-13502. DOI: 10.1074/jbc.M114.549832

[93] Fu C-CR, Shek E, Fleitman JS, de Leung MC. Collagen Containing Ophthalmic Formulation, Eur. Patent 90119626.1. Munich: European Patent Office; 1990

[94] Ghica MV, Albu MG, Popa L, Leca M, Brăzdaru L, Cotruț C, et al. Drug delivery systems based on collagen-tannic acid matrices. Revue Roumaine de Chimie. 2009;**54**(11):1103-1110

[95] Xeroudaki M, Thangavelu M, Lennikov A, Ratnayake A, Bisevac J, Petrovski G, et al. A porous collagen-based hydrogel and implantation method for corneal stromal regeneration and sustained local drug delivery. Scientific Reports. 2020;**10**:16936. DOI: 10.1038/ s41598-020-73730-9

[96] Ramírez OJ, Alvarez S, Contreras-Kallens P, Barrera NP, Aguayo S, Schuh CMAP. Type I collagen hydrogels as a delivery matrix for royal jelly derived extracellular vesicles. Drug Delivery. 2020;**27**(1):1308-1318. DOI: 10.1080/10717544.2020.1818880

[97] Dharunya G, Duraipandy N, Lakra R, Korapatti SK, Jayavel R, Kira MS. Curcumin cross-linked collagen aerogels with controlled anti-proteolytic and pro-angiogenic efficacy. Biomedical Materials. 2016;**11**:045011. DOI: 10.1088/1748-6041/11/4/045011

[98] Chuysinuan P, Chimnoi N, Reuk-Ngam N, Khlaychan P, Makarasen A, Wetprasit N, et al. Development of gelatin hydrogel pads incorporated with *Eupatorium adenophorum* essential oil as antibacterial wound dressing. Polymer Bulletin. 2018;**76**:701-724. DOI: 10.1007/s00289-018-2395-x

[99] Bettini S, Bonfrate V, Syrgiannis Z, Sannino A, Salvatore L, Madaghiele M, et al. Biocompatible collagen paramagnetic scaffold for controlled drug release. Biomacromolecules. 2015;**16**:2599-2608. DOI: 10.1021/acs.biomac.5b00829

[100] Reis LA, Chiu LL, Liang Y, Hyunh K, Momen A, Radisic M. A peptide-modified chitosan–collagen hydrogel for cardiac cell culture and delivery. Acta Biomaterialia. 2012;**8**:1022-1036

[101] Mei E, Li S, Song J, Xing R, Li Z, Yan X. Self-assembling collagen/alginate hybrid hydrogels for combinatorial photothermal and immuno tumor therapy. Colloids and Surfaces A: Physicochemical and Engineering Aspects. 2019;**577**:570-575. DOI: 10.1016/j.colsurfa.2019.06.023

[102] Choi M, Chung JH, Cho Y, Hong BY, Hong J. Nano-film modification of collagen hydrogels for controlled growth factor release. Chemical Engineering Science. 2015;**137**:626-630. DOI: 10.1016/j.ces.2015.07.011

[103] Choi D, Heo J, Park JH, Jo Y, Jeong H, Chang M, et al. Nano-film coatings onto collagen hydrogels with desired drug release. Journal of Industrial and Engineering Chemistry. 2016;**36925**:326-333. DOI: 10.1016/j.jiec.2016.02.023

[104] Djavid GE, Tabaie SM, Tajali SB, Totounchi M, Farhoud A, Fateh M, et al. Application of a collagen matrix dressing on a neuropathic diabetic foot ulcer: A randomised control trial. Journal of Wound Care. 2020;**2**(29,Sup3):S13-S18. DOI: 10.12968/jowc.2020.29.Sup3.S13

[105] Nguyen CH, Vu MQ, Phan TT, Vu TQ, Vo QA, Bach GL, et al. Novel pH-sensitive hydrogel beads based on carrageenan and fish scale collagen for allopurinol drug delivery. Journal of Polymers and the Environment. 2020;**28**:1795-1810. DOI: 10.1007/s10924-020-01727-6

[106] Wang X, Ronsin O, Gravez B, Farman N, Baumberger T, Jaisser F, et al. Nanostructured dense collagen-polyester composite hydrogels as amphiphilic platforms for drug delivery. Advanced Science. 2021;**18**(8):2004213. DOI: 10.1002/advs.202004213

[107] Li M, Han M, Sun Y, Hua Y, Chen G, Zhang L. Oligoarginine mediated collagen/chitosan gel composite for cutaneous wound healing. International Journal of Biological Macromolecules. 2019;**122**:1120-1127. DOI: 10.1016/j.ijbiomac.2018.09.061

[108] Chiu LL, Radisic M. Controlled release of thymosin β4 using collagen–chitosan composite hydrogels promotes epicardial cell migration and angiogenesis. Journal of Controlled

Release. 2011;**155**:376-385. DOI: 10.1016/j.jconrel.2011.05.026

[109] Davidson BS, Izzo F, Cromeens DM, Stephens LC, Siddik ZH, Curley SA. Collagen matrix cisplatin prevents local tumor growth after margin-positive resection. Journal of Surgical Research. 1995;**58**:618-624

[110] Ning S, Trisler K, Brown DM, Yu NY, Kanekal S, Lundsten MJ, et al. Intratumoral radioimmunotherapy of a human colon cancer xenograft using a sustained-release gel. Radiotherapy and Oncology. 1996;**39**:179-189

[111] Kanekal S, Sahai A, Jones RE, Brown D. Enhanced retention of ^{195m}Pt-cisplatin in murine tumors with a novel injectable sustained release drug delivery system. Pharmaceutical Research. 1995;**12**:S-228

[112] Slavin J, Nash JR, Kingsnorth AN. Effect of transforming growth factor beta and basic fibroblast growth factor on steroid impaired healing intestinal wound. British Journal of Surgery. 1992; **79**:69-72

[113] Weiner AL, Carpenter-Green SS, Soehngen EC, Lenk RP, Popescu MC. Liposome–collagen gel matrix: A novel sustained drug delivery system. Journal of Pharmaceutical Sciences. 1985;**74**: 922-925

[114] Pajean M, Herbage D. Effect of collagen on liposome permeability. International Journal of Pharmaceutics. 1993;**91**:209-216

[115] Fan X, Liang Y, Cui Y, Li F, Sun Y, Yang J, et al. Development of tilapia collagen and chitosan composite hydrogels for nanobody delivery. Colloids Surface B Biointerfaces. 2020; **195**:111261. DOI: 10.1016/j.colsurfb.2020.111261

[116] Wong FSY, Tsang KK, Chu AMW, Chan BP, Yao KM, Lo ACY. Injectable cell-encapsulating composite alginate-collagen platform with inducible termination switch for safer ocular drug delivery. Biomaterials. 2019;**201**:53-67. DOI: 10.1016/j.biomaterials.2019.01.032

[117] Bradley WG, Wilkes GL. Some mechanical property considerations of reconstituted collagen for drug release supports. Biomaterials, Medical Devices, and Artificial Organs. 1977;**5**:159-175

[118] McNamara TF, Ramamurthy NS, Golub LM. Non-Antibacterial Tetracycline Compositions Possessing Anti-Collagenolytic Properties and Methods of Preparing and Using Same. US Patent 4935412. Alexandria: US Patent and trademark office; 1990

[119] Minabe M, Takeuchi K, Tamura K, Hori T, Umemoto T. Subgingival administration of tetracycline on a collagen film. Journal of Periodontology. 1989;**60**:552-556

[120] Song S-Z, Morawiecki A, Pierce GF, Pitt CG. Collagen Film for Sustained Delivery of Proteins, Eur. Patent 92305467.3. Munich: European Patent Office; 1992

[121] Friess W, Lee G, Groves MJ. Insoluble collagen matrices for prolonged delivery of proteins. Pharmaceutical Development & Technology. 1996;**1**:185-193

[122] Gil CBS, Gil VSB, Carvalho SM, Silva GR, Magalhães JT, Rodrigo L, et al. Recycled collagen films as biomaterials for controlled drug delivery. New Journal of Chemistry. 2016;**40**: 8502-8510. DOI: 10.1039/C6NJ00674D

[123] Langasco R, Cadeddu B, Formato M, Lepedda AJ, Cossu M, Giunchedi P, et al. Natural collagenic skeleton of

marine sponges in pharmaceutics: Innovative biomaterial for topical drug delivery. Materials Science and Engineering: C. 2017;**70**:710-720. DOI: 10.1016/j.msec.2016.09.041

[124] Lee YI, Lee SG, Kim E, Jung I, Suk J, Kim J, et al. Anti-aging effect of an oral disintegrating collagen film: A prospective, single-arm study. International Journal of Dermatology. 2022;**61**(1):54-61. DOI: 10.1111/ijd.15675

[125] Walczak M, Michalska-Sionkowska M, Kaczmarek B, Sionkowska A. Surface and antibacterial properties of thin films based on collagen and thymol. Materials Today Communications. 2020;**22**: 100949. DOI: 10.1016/j.mtcomm.2020. 100949

[126] Skopinska-Wisniewska J, Sionkowska A, Kaminska A, Kaznica A, Jachimiak R, Drewa T. Surface characterization of collagen/elastin based biomaterials for tissue regeneration. Applied Surface Science. 2009;**255**(9):8286-8292

[127] Cascone MC, Sim B, Downes S. Blends of synthetic and natural polymers as drug delivery systems for growth hormone. Biomaterials. 1995;**16**:569-574

[128] Hong YJ, Chun J-S, LeeW-K. Association of collagen with calcium phosphate promoted osteogenic responses of osteoblast-like MG63 cells. Colloids and Surfaces B: Biointerfaces. 2011;**83**(2):245-253

[129] Park JC, Hwang YS, Lee JE, Park KD, Matsumura K, Hyon SH, et al. Type I atelocollagen grafting onto ozone-treated polyurethane films: Cell attachment, proliferation, and collagen synthesis. Journal of Biomedical Materials Research. 2000;**52**:669-677. DOI: 10.1002/1097-4636(20001215)52:4 <669::aid-jbm11>3.0.co;2-u

[130] Jana P, Mitra T, Selvaraj TKR, Gnanamani A, Kundu PP. Preparation of guar gum scaffold film grafted with ethylenediamine and fish scale collagen, crosslinked with ceftazidime for wound healing application. Carbohydrate Polymers. 2016;**153**(20):573-581. DOI: 10.1016/j.carbpol.2016.07.053

[131] Chen M, Huang Y-Q, Cao H, Liu Y, Guo H, Chen LS, et al. Collagen/chitosan film containing biotinylated glycol chitosan nanoparticles for localized drug delivery. Colloids and Surfaces B: Biointe rfaces. 2015;**128**:339-346. DOI: 10.1016/ j.colsurfb.2015.02.024

[132] Martino AD, Drannikov A, Surgutskaia NS, Ozaltin K, Postnikov PS, Marina TE, et al. Chitosan-collagen based film for controlled delivery of a combination of short life anesthetics. International Journal of Biological Mac romolecules. 2019;**140**:1183-1193. DOI: 10.1016/j.ijbiomac.2019.08.228

[133] Michalska-Sionkowska M, Kaczmarek B, Walczak M, Sionkowska A. Antimicrobial activity of new materials based on the blends of collagen/chitosan/hyaluronic acid with gentamicin sulfate addition. Materials Sc ience and Engineering: C. 2018;**86**: 103-108. DOI: 10.1016/j.msec.2018.01.005

[134] Tanum J, Heo J, Hong J. Spontaneous biomacromolecule absorption and long-term release by graphene oxide. ACS Omega. **2018**;*3*(*5*): 5903-5909. DOI: 10.1021/acsomega. 8b00537

[135] Yaşayan G, Karaca G, Akgüner ZP, Öztürk AB. Chitosan/collagen composite films as wound dressings encapsulating allantoin and lidocaine hydrochloride. International Journal of Polymeric Materials and Polymeric Biomaterials. 2020;**70**(9):623-635. DOI: 10.1080/ 00914037.2020.1740993

[136] Liu T, Dan W, Dan N, Liu X, Liu X, Peng X. A novel grapheme oxide-modified collagen-chitosan bio-film for controlled growth factor release in wound healing applications. Materials Science and Engineering: C Materials for Biological Applications. 2017;77:202-211. DOI: 10.1016/j.msec.2017.03.256

[137] Chen DW, Hsu Y-H, Liao J-Y, Liu S-J, Chen J-K, Ueng SW-N. Sustainable release of vancomycin, gentamicin and lidocaine from novel electrospun sandwich-structured PLGA/collagen nanofibrous membranes. International Journal of Pharmaceutics. 2012;**430**:335-341. DOI: 10.1016/j.ijpharm.2012.04.010

[138] Thacharodi D. Collagen-chitosan composite membranes controlled transdermal delivery of nifedipine and propranolol hydrochloride. International Journal of Pharmaceutics. 1996;**134**: 239-241. DOI: 10.1016/0378-5173(96) 04453-5

[139] Thacharodi D, Rao KP. Rate-controlling biopolymer membranes as transdermal delivery systems for nifedipine: Development and in vitro evaluations. Biomaterials. 1996;**13**: 1307-1311

[140] Lozeau LD, Grosha J, Kole D, Prifti F, Dominko T, Camesano TA, et al. Collagen tethering of synthetic human antimicrobial peptides cathelicidin LL37 and its effects on antimicrobial activity and cytotoxicity. Acta Biomaterialia. 2017;**52**:9-20. DOI: 10.1016/j.actbio. 2016.12.047

[141] Elangovan S, D'Mello SR, Hong L, Ross RD, Allamargot C, Dawson DV, et al. The enhancement of bone regeneration by gene activated matrix encoding for platelet derived growth factor. Biomaterials. 2014;**35**:737-747. DOI: 10.1016/j.biomaterials.2013.10.021

[142] Barroso T, Viveiros R, Casimiro T, Aguiar-Ricardo A. Development of dual-responsive chitosan–collagen scaffolds for pulsatile release of bioactive molecules. Journal of Supercritical Fluids. 2014;**94**:102-112. DOI: 10.1016/ j.supflu.2014.07.005

[143] Intaraprasit S, Faikrua SA, Viyoch J. Efficacy evaluation of the fibroblast-seeded collagen/ chitosan scaffold on application in skin tissue engineering. Science. Asia. 2012;**38**:268-277. DOI: 10.2306/scienceasia1513-1874.2012. 38.268

[144] Mao Z, Shi H, Guo R, Ma L, Gao C, Han C, et al. Enhanced angiogenesis of porous collagen scaffolds by incorporation of TMC/DNA complexes encoding vascular endothelial growth factor. Acta Biomaterialia. 2009;**5**:2983-2994. DOI: 10.1016/j.actbio.2009.04.004

[145] Kato A, Miyaji H, Ishizuka R, Tokunaga K, Inoue K, Kosen Y, et al. Combination of root surface modification with BMP-2 and collagen hydrogel scaffold implantation for periodontal healing in beagle dogs. Open Dentistry Journal. 2015;**30**(9):52-59. DOI: 10.2174/1874210601509010052

[146] Moshiri A, Shahrezaee M, Shekarchi AK. Three-dimensional porous gelapin–simvastatin scaffolds promoted bone defect healing in rabbits. Calcified Tissue International. 2015; **96**:552-564. DOI: 10.1007/s00223-015-9981-9

[147] Karri VVSR, Kuppusamy G, Talluri SV, Mannemala SS, Kollipara R, Wadhwani AD, et al. Curcumin loaded chitosan nanoparticles impregnated into collagen-alginate scaffolds for diabetic wound healing. International Journal of Biological Macromolecules. 2016;**93**: 1519-1529. DOI: 10.1016/j.ijbiomac. 2016.05.038

[148] Mahmoud AA, Salama AH. Norfloxacin-loaded collagen/chitosan scaffolds for skin reconstruction: Preparation, evaluation and in-vivo wound healing assessment. European Journal of Pharmaceutical Sciences. 2016;**83**:155-165. DOI: 10.1016/j.ejps.2015.12.026

[149] Chow JP, Simionescu DT, Warner H, Wang B, Patnaik SS, Liao J, et al. Mitigation ofdiabetes-related complications in implanted collagen and elastin scaffolds using matrix-binding polyphenol. Biomaterials. 2013;**34**: 685-695. DOI: 10.1016/j.biomaterials.2012.09.081

[150] López-Noriega A, Ruiz-Hernández E, Quinlan E, Storm G, Hennink WE, O'Brien FJ. Thermally triggered release of apro-osteogenic peptide from a functionalized collagen-based scaffold using thermo- sensitive liposomes. Journal of Controlled Release. 2014;**187**: 158-166. DOI: 10.1016/j.jconrel.2014.05.043

[151] Cao H, Chen M-M, Liu Y-Y, Huang Y-Q, Wang J-H, Chen J-D, et al. Fish collagen-based scaffold containing PLGA microspheres for controlled growth factor delivery in skin tissue engineering. Colloids and Surfaces B: Biointerfaces. 2015;**136**:1098-1106. DOI: 10.1016/j.colsurfb.2015.10.022

[152] Urello MA, Kiick KL, Sullivan MO. ECM turnoverstimulated gene delivery through collagen-mimetic peptide-plasmid integration in collagen. Acta Biomaterialia. 2017;**62**:167-178. DOI: 10.1016/j.actbio.2017.08.038

[153] do Amaral RJFC, Zayed NMA, Pascu EI, Cavanagh B, Hobbs C, Santarella F, et al. Functionalising collagen-based scaffolds with platelet-rich plasma for enhanced skin wound healing potential. Frontiers in Bioengineering and Biotechnology. 2019; **3**(7):371. DOI: 10.3389/fbioe.2019.00371

[154] Lee D, Wufuer M, Kim I, Choi TH, Kim BJ, Jung HG, et al. Sequential dual-drug delivery of BMP-2 and alendronate from hydroxyapatite-collagen scaffolds for enhanced bone regeneration. Scientific Reports. 2021;**12**(11):746. DOI: 10.1038/s41598-020-80608-3

[155] Rezaii M, Oryan S, Javeri A. Curcumin nanoparticles incorporated collagen-chitosan scffold promotes cutaneous wound healing through regulation of TGF-β1/Smad7 gene expression. Materials Science & Engineering: C. 2019;**98**:347-357. DOI: 10.1016/j.msec.2018.12.143

[156] Marks MG, Doillon C, Silver FH. Effects of fibroblasts and basic fibroblast growth factor on facilitation of dermal wound healing by type I collagen matrices. Journal of Biomedical Materials Research. 1991;**25**:683-696

[157] Kenley RA, Yim K, Abrams J, Ron E, Turek T, Marden LJ, et al. Biotechnology and bone graft substitutes. Pharmaceutical Research. 1993;**10**:1393-1401

[158] Fujimura K, Bessho K, Kusumoto K, Ogawa Y, Iizuka T. Experimental studies on bone inducing activity of composites of a telopeptide type I collagen as a carrier for ectopic induction by rhBMP-2. Biochemical and Biophysical Research Communications. 1995;**208**:316-322

[159] Horisaka Y, Okamoto Y, Matsumoto N, Yoshimura Y, Hirano A, Nishida M, et al. Histological changes of implanted collagen material during bone induction. Journal of Biomedical Materials Research. 1994;**28**:97-103

[160] Wachol-Drewek Z, Pfeiffer M, Scholl E. Comparative investigation of

drug delivery of collagen implants saturated in antibiotic solutions and a sponge containing gentamicin. Biomaterials. 1996;**17**:1733-1738

[161] Peng YM, Alberts DS, Graham V, Surwit EA, Weiner S, Meyskens FL. Cervical tissue uptake of all-*trans*-retinoic acid delivered via a collagen sponge–cervical cap delivery device in patients with cervical dyplasia. Investigational New Drugs. 1986;**4**:245-249

[162] Barbaresso RC, Rau I, Zgârian RG, Meghea A, Ghica MV. Niflumic acid-collagen delivery systems used as anti-inflammatory drugs and analgesics in dentistry. Comptes Rendus Chimie. 2014;**17**:12-17. DOI: 10.1016/j.crci.2013.07.007

[163] Chia CLK, Shelat VG, Low W, George S, Rao J. The use of Collatamp® G, local gentamicin-collagen sponge, in reducing wound infection. International Surgery. 2014;**99**:565-570. DOI: 10.9738/INTSURG-D-13-00171.1

[164] Bhakta G, Lim ZXH, Rai B, Lin T, Hui JH, Preswich GD, et al. The influence of collagen and hyaluronan matrices on the delivery and bioactivity of bone morphogenetic protein-2 and ectopic bone formation. Acta Biomaterialia. 2013;**9**(11):9098-9106. DOI: 10.1016/j.actbio.2013.07.008

[165] Wen F, Chang S, Toh YC, Teoh SH, Yu H. Development of poly (lactic-coglycolicacid)-collagen scaffolds for tissue engineering. Materials Science and Engineering: C. 2007;**27**(2):285-292

[166] Alagha A, Nourallah A, Hariri S. Characterization of dexamethasone loaded collagen-chitosan sponge and in vitro release study. Journal of Drug De livery Science and Technology. 2020;**55**: 101449. DOI: 10.1016/j.jddst.2019.101449

[167] Schlapp M, Friess W. Collagen/PLGA microparticle composites for local controlled delivery of gentamicin. Journa l of Pharmaceutical Sciences. 2003;**92**: 2145-2151. DOI: 10.1002/jps.10460

[168] David G, Bargan AI, Drobota M, Bele A, Rosca I. Comparative investigation of collagen-based hybrid 3D structures for potential biomedical applications. Materials. 2021;**14**(12): 3313. DOI: 10.3390/ma14123313

[169] Helary C, Abed A, Mosser G, Louedec L, Letourneur D, Coradin T, et al. Evaluation of dense collagen matrices as medicated wound dressing for the treatment of cutaneous chronic wounds. Biomaterials Science. 2015;**3**:373-382. DOI: 10.1039/C4BM00370E

[170] De-Souza R, Zahedi P, Allen CJ, Piquette-Miller M. Polymeric drug delivery systems for localized cancer chemotherapy. Drug Delivery. 2010; **2010**(17):365-375. DOI: 10.31090037 62854

[171] Orsi S, Capua De A, Guarnieri D, Marasco D, Netti PA. Cell recruitment and transfection in gene activated collagen matrix. Biomaterials. 2010;**31**: 570-576. DOI: 10.1016/j.biomaterials.2009.09.054

[172] Li J, Mooney DJ. Designing hydrogels for controlled drug delivery. Nature Review Materials. 2016;**1**:16071. DOI: 10.1038/natrevmats.2016.71

[173] Davidenko N, Campbell JJ, Thian ES, Watson CJ, Cameron RE. Collagen–hyaluronic acid scaffolds for adipose tissue engineering. Acta Biomaterialia. 2010;**6**(10):3957-3968

[174] Stadlinger B, Pilling E, Huhle M, Mai R, Bierbaum S, Scharnweber D, et al. Evaluation of osseointegration of dental implants coated with collagen,

chondroitin sulphate and BMP-4: An animal study. International Journal of Oral and Maxillofacial Surgery. 2008; **37**(1):54-59

[175] Stamov D, Grimmer M, Salchert K, Pompe T, Werner C. Heparin intercalation into reconstituted collagen I fibrils: Impact on growth kinetics and morphology. Biomaterials. 2008; **29**(1):1-14

[176] Gotterbarm T, Richter W, Jung M, Vilei SB, Mainil-Varlet P, Yamashita T, et al. An in vivo study of a growth-factor enhanced, cell free, two-layered collagen–tricalcium phosphate in deep osteochondral defects. Biomaterials. 2006;**27**(18):3387-3395

[177] Wong HL, Wang MX, Cheung PT, Yao KM, Chan BP. A 3D collagen microsphere culture system for GDNF-secreting HEK293 cells with enhanced protein productivity. Biomaterials. 2007; **28**:5369-5380. DOI: 10.1016/j.bio materials.2007.08.016

[178] Solorio L, Zwolinkski C, Lund AW, Farrell MJ, Stegemann JP. Gelatin microspheres crosslinked with genipin for local delivery of growth factors. Journal of Tissue Engineering and Regenerative Medicine. 2010;**4**:514-523. DOI: 10.1002/term.267

[179] Huang Z, Feng Q, Yu B, Li S. Biomimetic properties of an injectable chitosan/nano-hydroxyapatite/collagen composite. Materials Science & Engineering: C. 2011;**31**:683-687. DOI: 10.1016/j.msec.2010.12.014

[180] Lee M, Lo ACY, Cheung P, Wong D, Chan BP. Drug carrier systems based on collagen–alginate composite structures for improving the performance of GDNF-secreting HEK293 cells. Biomaterials. 2009;**30**: 1214-1221. DOI: 10.1016/j.biomaterials. 2008.11.017

[181] Mansouri V, Salehi M, Omrani MD, Niknam Z, Ardeshirylajimi A. Collagen-alginate microspheres as a 3D culture system for mouse embryonic stem cells differentiation to primordial germ cells. Biologicals. 2017;**48**:114-120. DOI: 10.1016/j.biologicals.2017.04.003

[182] Rössler B. Entwicklung und Untersuchung von Kollagen mikropartikelnalsWirkstoffträger in Hydrogelen am Beispiel all-*trans* Retinol [Thesis]. Frankfurt: University of Frankfurt; 1993

[183] Gebhardt BM, Kaufman HE. Collagen as a delivery system for hydrophobic drugs: Studies with cyclosporine. Journal of Ocular Pharmacology and Therapeutics. 1995; **11**:319-327

[184] Gebhardt BM, Varnell ED, Kaufman HE. Cyclosporine in collagen particles: Corneal penetration and suppression of allograft rejection. Journal of Ocular Pharmacology and Therapeutics. 1995;**11**:509-517

[185] Berthold A, Cremer K, Kreuter J. Collagen microparticles: Carriers for glucocorticosteroids. European Journal of Pharmaceutics and Biopharmaceutics. 1998;**45**:23-29

[186] Calejo MT, Almeida AJ, Fernandes AI. Exploring a new jellyfish collagen in the production of microparticles for protein delivery. Journal of Microencapsulation. 2012;**29**: 520-531. DOI: 10.3109/02652048.2012. 665089

[187] Rössler B, Kreuter J, Ross G. Effect of collagen microparticles on the stability of retinol and its absorption into hairless

mouse skin in vitro. Die Pharmazie. 1994;**49**:175-179

[188] Kreuter J, Scherer D, Müller W, Roreger M. VerfahrenzurHerstellung von Kollagenpartikeln und ihreVerwendungalsWirkstofftra, German Patent 4038887. Munich: German Patent and Trademark Office; 1990

[189] Zugravu MV, Smith RA, Reves BT, Jennings JA, Cooper JO, Haggard WO, et al. Physical properties and in vitro evaluation of collagen–chitosan–calcium phosphate microparticle-based scaffolds for bone tissue regeneration. Journal of Biomaterials Applications. 2013;**28**(4): 566-579. DOI: 10.1177/0885328212465662

[190] Vardar E, Larsson HM, Allazetta S, Engelhardt EM, Pinnagoda K, Vythilingam G, et al. Microfluidic production of bioactive fibrin micro-beads embedded in crosslinked collagen used as an injectable bulking agent for urinary incontinence treatment. Acta Biomaterialia. 2018;**67**:156-166. DOI: 10.1016/j.actbio.2017.11.034

[191] Nicklas M, Schatton W, Heinemann S, Hanke T, Kreuter J. Preparation and characterization of marine sponge collagen nanoparticles and employment for the transdermal delivery of 17b-estradiol-hemihydrate. Drug Development & Industrial Pharmacy. 2009;**35**:1035-1042. DOI: 10.1080/03639040902755213

[192] Jahanban-Esfahlan R, Derakhshankhah H, Haghshenas B, Massoumi B, Abbasian M, Jaymand M. A bio-inspired magnetic natural hydrogel containing gelatin and alginate as a drug delivery system for cancer chemotherapy. International Journal of Biological Macromolecules. 2020;**156**: 438-445. DOI: 10.1016/j.ijbiomac.2020.04.074

[193] Anandhakumar S, Krishnamoorthy G, Ramkumar K, Raichur A. Preparation of collagen peptide functionalized chitosan nanoparticles by ionic gelation method: An effective carrier system for encapsulation and release of doxorubicin for cancer drug delivery. Materials Science & Engineering: C. 2017;**70**: 378-385. DOI: 10.1016/j.msec.2016.09.003

[194] Guo H, Hong Z, Yi R. Core-shell collagen peptide chelated calcium/calcium alginate nanoparticles from fish scales for calcium supplementation. Journal of Food Science. 2015;**80**:N1595-N1601. DOI: 10.1111/1750-3841.12912

[195] Choi J, Park H, Kim T, Jeong Y, Oh MH, Hyeon T, et al. Engineered collagen hydrogels for the sustained release of biomolecules and imaging agents: Promoting the growth of human gingival cells. International Journal of Nanomedicine. 2014;**9**(1):5189-5201. DOI: 10.2147/IJN.S71304

[196] Minakuchi Y, Takeshita F, Kosaka N, Sasaki H, Yamamoto Y, Kouno M, et al. Ochiya T. Atelocollagen-mediated synthetic small interfering RNA delivery for effective gene silencing *in vitro* and *in vivo*. Nucleic Acids Research. 2004; **32**(13):e109. DOI: 10.1093/nar/gnh093

[197] Saska S, Teixeira LN, De Castro-Raucci LMS, Scarel-Caminaga RM, Franchi LP, Dos Santos RA, et al. Nanocellulose-collagen-apatite composite associated with osteogenic growth peptide for bone regeneration. International Journal of Biological Macromolecules. 2017;**103**:467-476. DOI: 10.1016/j.ijbiomac.2017.05.086

[198] Sotome S, Uemura T, Kikuchi M, Chen J, Itoh S, Tanaka J, et al. Synthesis

and in vivo evaluation of a novel hydroxyapatite/collagen–alginate as a bone filler and a drug delivery carrier of bone morphogenetic protein. Materials Science & Engineering: C. 2004;**24**:341-347. DOI: 10.1016/j.msec.2003.12.003

[199] Schnell E, Klinkhammer K, Balzer S, Brook G, Klee D, Dalton P, et al. Guidance of glial cell migration and axonal growth on electrospun nanofibers of poly-ε-caprolactone and a collagen/poly-ε-caprolactone blend. Biomaterials. 2007;**28**(19):3012-3025

[200] Bloomfield SE, Miyata T, Dunn MW, Bueser N, Stenzel KH, Rubin AL. Soluble gentamicin ophthalmic inserts as a drug delivery system. Ophthalmology. 1978;**96**:885-887

[201] Punch PI, Costa ND, Edwards ME, Wilcox GE. The release of insoluble antibiotics from collagen ocular inserts in vitro and their insertion into the conjunctival sac of cattle. Journal of Veterinary Pharmacology and Therapeutics. 1987;**10**:37-42

[202] Rubin AL, Stenzel KH, Miyata T, White MJ, Dunn MW. Collagen as a vehicle for drug delivery. Journal of Clinical Pharmacology. 1973;**17**:309-312

[203] Poland DE, Kaufman HE. Clinical uses of collagen shields. Journal of Cataract Refractive Surgery. 1988;**14**:489-491

[204] Phinney RB, Schwartz SD, Lee DA, Mondino BJ. Collagen shield delivery of gentamicin and vancomycin. Archives of Ophthalmology. 1988;**106**:1599-1604

[205] Milani JK, Verbukh I, Pleyer U, Sumner H, Adamu SA, Halabi HP, et al. Collagen shields impregnated with gentamicin-dexamethasone as a potential drug delivery device. American Journal of Ophthalmology. 1993;**116**:622-627

[206] Dorigo MT, De Natale R, Miglioli PA. Collagen shields delivery of netilmicin: A study of ocular pharmacokinetics. Chemotherapy. 1995;**41**:1-4

[207] Mendicute J, Ondarra A, Eder F, Ostolaza JI, Salaberria M, Lamsfus JM. The use of collagen shields impregnated with amphotericin B to treat *aspergillus* keratomycosis. CLAO Journal. 1995;**21**:252-255

[208] Palmer RM, McDonald MB. A corneal lens/shield system to promote postoperative corneal epithelial healing. Journal of Cataract Refractive Surgery. 1995;**21**:125-126

[209] Finkelstein I, Trope GE, Meno IA, Rootsman D, Basu PK. Potential value of collagen shields as a subconjunctival depot release system. Current Eye Research. 1990;**90**:653-659

[210] Hwang DG, Stern WH, Hwang PH, MacGowan-Smith LA. Collagen shield enhancement of topical dexamethasone penetration. Archives of Ophthalmology. 1989;**107**:1375-1380

[211] Takeuchi K. Application of local drug delivery systems to periodontal therapy. Nihon-shishubyo-gakkai-kaishi. 1992;**34**:741-758

[212] Matsuoka J, Sakagami K, Shiozaki S, Uchida S, Fujiwara T, Gohchi A, et al. Development of an interleukin-2 slow delivery system. Transactions of the American Society for Artificial Internal Organs. 1988;**34**:729-731

[213] Fujioka Y, Takada Y. Collagen-based drug delivery system – development of minipellet system. Pharmaceutical Technology, Japan. 1991;**7**:402-409

[214] Zhou J, Cao C, Ma X, Lin J. Electrospinning of silk fibroin and collagen for vascular tissue engineering. International Journal of Biological Macromolecules. 2010;**47**(4):514-519

[215] Chen Y, Mak AFT, Wang M, Li J, Wong MS. PLLA scaffolds with biomimetic apatite coating and biomimetic apatite/collagen composite coating to enhance osteoblast-like cells attachment and activity. Surface and Coatings Technology. 2006;**201**(3–4): 575-580

[216] Nicklas M, Schatton W, Heinemann S, Hanke T, Kreuter J. Enteric coating derived from marine sponge collagen. Drug Development & Industrial Pharmacy. 2009;**35**:1384-1388. DOI: 10.3109/03639040902939239

[217] de Bruin AF, Gosselink MP, van der Harst E, Rutten HJ. Local application of gentamicin collagen implants in the prophylaxis of surgical site infections following gastrointestinal surgery: A review of clinical experience. Techniques in Coloproctology. 2010;**14**: 301-310. DOI: 10.1007/s10151-010-0593-0

[218] Friess W, Zhou W, Groves MJ. In vivo activity of collagen matrices containing PS1, an anti-neoplastic glycan, against murine sarcoma cells. Journal of Pharmacy and Pharmacology. 2011;**2**(3):121-124. DOI: 10.1111/j.2042-7158.1996.tb00573.x

[219] Sun X, Yang X, Song W, Ren L. Construction and evaluation of collagen-based corneal grafts using polycaprolactone to improve tension stress. ACS Omega. 2020;**145**(1): 674-682. DOI: 10.1021/acsomega.9b03297

[220] Lin Z, Wu T, Wang W, Li B, Wang M, Chen L, et al. Biofunctions of antimicrobial peptide-conjugated alginate/hyaluronic acid/collagen wound dressings promote wound healing of a mixed-bacteria-infected wound. International Journal of Biological Macromolecules. 2019;**140**:330-342. DOI: 10.1016/j.ijbiomac.2019.08.087

[221] Abdel-Mohsen AM, Frankova J, Abdel-Rahman RM, Salem AA, Sahffiee NM, Kubena I, et al. Chitosan-glucan complex hollow fibers reinforced collagen wound dressing embedded with aloe vera. II. Multifunctional properties to promote cutaneous wound healing. International Journal of Pharmaceutics. 2020;**582**:119349. DOI: 10.1016/j.ijpharm.2020.119349

[222] Dimatteo R, Darling NJ, Segura T. In situ forming injectable hydrogels for drug delivery and wound repair. Advanced Drug Delivery Reviews. 2018; **127**:167-184. DOI: 10.1016/j.addr.2018.03.007

[223] Zustiak SP, Leach JB. Hydrolytically degradable poly(ethylene glycol) hydrogel scaffolds with tunable degradation and mechanical properties. Biomacromolecules. 2010;**11**:1348-1357. DOI: 10.1021/bm100137q

[224] Narayanaswamy R, Torchilin VP. Hydrogels and their applications in targeted drug delivery. Molecules. 2019; **24**:E603. DOI: 10.3390/molecules24030603

[225] Ruskowitz RE, DeForest AC. Photoresponsive biomaterials for targeted drug delivery and 4D cell culture. Nature Reviews Materials. 2018; **3**:1-17. DOI: 10.1038/natrevmats2017.87

[226] Karki S, Kim H, Na S-J, Shin D, Jo K, Lee J. Thin films as an emerging platform for drug delivery. Asian Journal of Pharmaceutical Sciences. 2016;**11**: 559-574. DOI: 10.1016/j.ajps.2016.05.004

[227] Borges AF, Silva C, Coelho JF, Simões S. Oral films: Current status and future perspectives: I - Galenical development and quality attributes. Journal of Controlled Release. 2015;**206**: 1-19. DOI: 10.1016/j.jconrel.2015.03.006

[228] Castro PM, Fonte P, Sousa F, Madureira RA, Sarmento B, Pintado ME. Oral films as breakthrough tools for oral delivery of proteins/peptides. Journal of Controlled Release. 2015;**211**:63-73. DOI: 10.1016/j.jconrel.2015.05.258

[229] Zhang Q, Lu H, Kawazoe N, Chen G. Pore size effect of collagen scaffolds on cartilage regeneration. Acta Biomaterilia. 2014;**10**:2005-2013. DOI: 10.1016/j.actbio.2013.12.042

[230] Higuchi A, Ling Q-D, Hsu S-T, Umezawa A. Biomimetic cell culture proteins as extracellular matrices for stem cell differentiation. Chemical Reviews. 2012;**112**:4507-4540. DOI: 10.1021/cr3000169

[231] Berndt M, Li Y, Seyedhassantehrani N, Yao L. Fabrication and characterization of microspheres encapsulating astrocytes for neural regeneration. ACS Biomaterials Science & Engineering. 2017;**3**:1313-1321. DOI: 10.1021/acsbiomaterials.6b00229

[232] Yang C, Fang C. Microporous nano-hydroxyapatite/collagen/phosphatidylserine scaffolds embedding collagen microparticles for controlled drug delivery in bone tissue engineering. Materials Research. **2015;18(5)**:1077-1081. DOI: 10.1590/1516-1439.042115

[233] Padovani GC, Feitosa VP, Sauro S, Tay FR, Durán G, Paula AJ, et al. Advances in dental materials through nanotechnology: Facts, perspectives and toxicological aspects. Trends in Biotechnology. 2015;**33**:621-636. DOI: 10.1016/j.tibtech.2015.09.005

[234] DeFrates K, Markiewicz T, Gallo P, Rack A, Weyhmiller A, Jarmusik B, et al. Protein polymer-based nanoparticles: Fabrication and medical applications. International Journal of Molecular Sciences. 2018;**19**:E1717. DOI: 10.3390/ijms19061717

[235] Mandal A, Farhan MK, Sastry TP. Effect of reinforced Al_2O_3 nanoparticles on collagen nanobiocomposite from chrome-containing leather waste for biomedical applications. Clean Technologies & Environmental Policy. 2016;**18**:765-773. DOI: 10.1007/s10098-015-1045-3

[236] Srivatsan KV, Duraipandy N, Behum S, Lakra R, Ramamutrthy U, Saikorrapati P, et al. Effect of curcumin caged silver nanoparticle on collagen stabilization for biomedical applications. International Journal of Biological Macromolecules. 2015;**75**:306-315. DOI: 10.1016/j.ijbiomac.2015.01.050

[237] Saleh T, Ahmed E, Yu L, Hussein K, Park K-M, Lee Y-S, et al. Silver nanoparticles improve structural stability and biocompatibility of decellularized porcine liver. Artificial Cells, Nanomedicine & Biotechnology. 2018;**46**(2):273-284. DOI: 10.1080/21691401.2018.1457037

[238] Robin JB, Keys CL, Kaminski LA, Viana MA. The effect of collagen shields on rabbit corneal reepithelialization after chemical debridement. Investigative Ophthalmology & Visual Science. 1990; **31**:1294-1300

[239] Shaker GJ, Ueda S, LoCascio JA, Aquavella JV. Effect of collagen shield on cat corneal epithelial wound healing. Investigative Ophthalmology & Visual Science. 1989;**30**:1565-1568

[240] Sahithi B, Ansari SK, Hameeda SK, Sahithya G, Durga PM, Yogitha L. A

review on collagen based drug delivery systems. Indian Journal of Research in Pharmacy and Biotechnology. 2013;**1**(3): 461-468

[241] Fujioka K, Takada Y, Sato S, Miyata T. Novel delivery system for proteins using collagen as a carrier material: The minipellet. Journal of Controlled Release. 1995;**33**:307-315

[242] Maeda H, Sano A, Fujioka K. Profile of rhBMP-2 release from collagen minipellet and induction of ectopic bone formation. Drug Development and Industrial Pharmacy. 2004;**30**(5): 473-480. DOI: 10.1081/DDC-120037475

[243] Lofthouse S, Nagahara S, Sedgmen B, Barcham G, Brandon M, Sano A. The application of biodegradable collagen minipellets as vaccine delivery vehicles in mice and sheep. Vaccine. 2001; **19**(30):4318-4327. DOI: 10.1016/s0264-410x(01)00153-0

[244] Higaki M, Azechi Y, Takase T, Igarashi R, Nagahara S, Sano A, et al. Collagen minipellet as a controlled release delivery system for tetanus and diphtheria toxoid. Vaccine. 2001; **19**(23-24):3091-3096. DOI: 10.1016/s0264-410x(01)00039-1

Chapter 6

Collagen Based 3D Printed Scaffolds for Tissue Engineering

Sougata Ghosh, Bishwarup Sarkar, Ratnakar Mishra, Nanasaheb Thorat and Sirikanjana Thongmee

Abstract

Tissue grafting is mostly used for repair and replacement of severely damaged tissues, the key challenges are compatibility, availability of the grafts, complex surgical process and post-operative complications. Hence, additive technologies such as three-dimensional (3D) bioprinting have emerged as promising alternative for tissue engineering in order to ensure safety, compatibility, and rapid healing. The aim of this chapter is to give an elaborate account of 3D printed scaffolds for bone, cartilage, cardio-vascular and nerve tissue engineering. Various components such as polycaprolactone, poly (lactic-co-glycolic acid), and β-tricalcium phosphate, bioglass 45S5, and nano-hydroxyapatite are combined with collagen and its derivatives to achieve specific pore size in the scaffolds for effective restoration of the defects of soft or hard tissues. Likewise, proanthocyanidin, oxidized hyaluronic acid, methacrylated gelatin, are used in collagen based 3D printed scaffolds for cartilage tissue engineering. Bioink with collagen as active component is also used for developing cardio-vascular implants with recellularizing properties. Collagen in combination with silk fibroin, chitosan, heparin sulphate and others are ideal for fabrication of elastic nerve guidance conduits. In view of the background, collagen-supplemented hydrogels can revolutionize future biomedical approaches for the development of complex scaffolds for tissue engineering.

Keywords: biomaterial, collagen, scaffolds, 3D printing, tissue engineering, regenerative medicine

1. Introduction

Biomedical application of nanotechnology has revolutionized tissue engineering as it can generate efficient biocompatible scaffolds with tuneable physico-chemical properties. Controllable biodegradability is one of the most important aspects as it supports the cells to produce extracellular matrix and promote effective healing. Likewise, adjustable pore structures of the scaffolds provides attractive site for loading drugs for resisting post-surgical infections and promoting cell attachment and colonization. Excellent biomechanical properties obtained by rational selection of the bioink help to mimic the tissue microenvironment and provide load bearing capacity to the tissue after repair [1]. Adherence of cells, proliferation and induction of osteogenic differentiation is higher when the total porosity of the 3D printed surfaces are more than 90% [2, 3]. Hence, such scaffolds with architectural specificity to the desired tissue like bone, cartilage, heart or nerves is immensely critical during implantation in order to ensure regeneration of the new tissue followed by repair [4].

Complete healing in traumatic injury is often a challenge that requires complicated surgical procedures which are often associated with failures and post-surgical infections. Till date bone grafting using autografts, allografts, xenografts, and synthetic bone grafts are employed for fixing the injury [5, 6]. However, the factors critical for success of grafting are the optimal size, shape, biomaterial and the anatomical structure of the bone defects. Thus, 3D printed scaffolds or synthetic bone grafts are considered more feasible due to their tuneable mechanical properties identical to the original bone tissue, and ease of rapid re-vascularization [7].

Weakening and gradual damage to cartilage may also lead to joint injury. Likewise, sudden traumatic injury, formation of lesions and developmental defects may also result is degradation of cartilage and impairment of its function [8]. In the United States alone, it is estimated that around 200,000–300,000 patients have undergone cartilage surgery [9]. It is important to note that the articular cartilage is non-neural, lymphatic, and avascular, having very low self-regenerating capacity [10]. Hence 3D printing mediated fabrication of scaffolds for repair or replacement is thought to be one of the most preferable technologies for cartilage tissue engineering [11]. Similarly, in treating cardiac dysfunctions, it is essential to maintain and mimic the cardiovascular anatomy while fixing the heart defects using tissue engineered vascular grafts (TEVGs). The 3D printing has tremendously helped to fabricate patient- and operation-specific vascular grafts [12]. Further, growing cases of neurodegenerative diseases also require effective therapeutic interventions, which are ideal for axonal regeneration and functional recovery for brain and spinal cord injury (SCI). Neuroregenerative scaffolds developed by 3D printing are considered as innovative materials that mainly focus on providing supportive substrates to guide axons and break the physical and chemical barriers, thereby promoting healing [13].

Collagen type 1 is most favorable for microextrusion based 3D bioprinting of biodegradable and biosorbable scaffolds. Collagen type 1 is the most predominant protein in the extracellular and intercellular matrix, constituting 20–30% of the vertebrate connective tissue, alongside hyaluronic acid (HA). Most importantly, the biocompatibility and low antigenicity of the collagen is attributed to the repeating motifs formed by the alpha chain of hydroxyproline-proline-glycine [14]. Collagen provides highly porous structure and hence permeability which in turn facilitates adhesion, migration, differentiation in addition to the regulation of the cellular morphology [15, 16].

This chapter highlights the collagen based 3D printed scaffolds with their attractive properties such as hydrophilicity, biodegradability, permeability, plasticity and biocompatibility critical for tissue engineering.

2. Collagen based 3D bioprinting of tissues

Biomaterials composed of collagen as listed in **Table 1** are considered ideal substrate for 3D printing mediated fabrication of scaffolds for tissue engineering purposes [32]. However, simulation of the tissue microenvironment is crucial to mimic the physical and morphological properties of the native tissues in order to

Tissue	Biomaterials		Reference
Bone	polycaprolactone (PCL), poly (lactic-co-glycolic acid) (PLGA), and β-tricalcium phosphate (β-TCP), atelocollagen	circular calvarial defects in male Sprague–Dawley rats	[17]
Bone	calcium phosphate, Phosphoric acid, collagen	critically sized murine femoral defect	[18]
Bone	Bioglass 45S5 (BG), methacrylated collagen (CMA)	human mesenchymal stem cells	[19]
Bone	mesoporous bioactive glass (BG) microspheres with 4% molar percentage of strontium, Type I collagen	simulated body fluid (SBF)	[20]
Bone	rod-like nano-hydroxyapatite particles embedded in a type I collagen matrix	—	[21]
Cartilage	collagen, oligomeric proanthocyanidin, oxidized hyaluronic acid	rat bone marrow mesenchymal stem cells (rBMSCs), bone defects in skulls of the Sprague Dawley (SD) rat	[22]
Cartilage	methacrylated gelatin (GelMA), nanohydroxyapatite (nHA)	bone marrow mesenchymal stem cells (BMSCs), rabbit osteochondral defect	[23]
Cartilage	crude collagen extracted from tendons of skeletally mature rat tails	primary meniscal fibrochondrocytes	[24]
Heart valve	gelatin support gel 3D printed with Lifeink® 200	subcutaneous implantation in Sprague–Dawley rats	[25]
Neonatal scale human heart	gelated collagen	human stem cell–derived cardiomyocytes	[12]
Cardiac tissue	gelatin, gum arabic microparticles, rat collagen-I	human induced pluripotent stem cells (hiPSC)-cardiomyocytes	[26]
Nerve	collagen, silk fibroin	neural stem cells (NSCs), spinal cord injury (SCI) in Sprague–Dawley rats	[27]
Peripheral nerve	poly-lactic acid (PLA), collagen	PC-12 cells, Schwann cells, and primary chick dorsal root ganglia	[28]
Elastic nerve guidance conduits (NGCs)	poly(lactide-*co*-caprolactone) (PLCL), collagen hydrogel	sciatic nerve injury models in rats	[29]
Neural tissue	VEGF-releasing fibrin gel, Type I collagen	C17.2 cells	[30]
Axon	chitosan, collagen	spinal cord injury (SCI) in rats	[31]
Spinal cord	heparin sulfate, collagen	neural stem cells (NSCs) from embryonic day 14 (E14) brains, spinal cord injury (SCI) in rats	[13]

Table 1.
Collagen based biomaterials for 3D printed tissues.

ensure proper restoration and replacement. The following section elaborates various advances of 3D bioprinting with collagen for tissue engineering.

2.1 Bone

Collagen based scaffolds are widely used for bone tissue engineering. Hwang et al. (2017) fabricated bone grafts employing 3D printing using a composite of polycaprolactone (PCL), poly (lactic-co-glycolic acid) (PLGA), and β-tricalcium phosphate (β-TCP) mixed in a ratio of 4:4:2 [17]. **Figure 1** shows the scanning electron microscope (SEM) images of the bone grafts. The bone graft developed by solid freeform fabrication (SFF) technique were further mixed with 3% atelocollagen and poured into a mold and incubated at 37°C for 15 min followed by deep freezing for 6 h and freeze drying for 12 h. The collagen based biomaterial was then immersed in ethanol/water (90% v/v) co-solvent containing 50 mM of 1-ethyl-3-(3-dimethyaminopropyl) carbodiimide (EDC) and 20 mM of N-hydroxysuccinimide (NHS) for 24 h at room temperature for effective cross-linking. Each cross-linked collagen block had a diameter and height of 8 mm and 2 mm, respectively. Circular calvarial defects of 8 mm diameter were created by removal of periosteum in male Sprague–Dawley rats. The PCL/PLGA/β-TCP composite block bone grafts were implanted into the defect cites. Interestingly the bone grafts were surrounded by fibrous connective tissues. Subtle bone formation was noted while infiltration of the giant cell and inflammatory cells were seen. However, after eight weeks both neovascularization and new bone formation were noted around the bone grafts. It was speculated that these novel PCL/PLGA/β-TCP composite block bone grafts may be considered as an alternative to synthetic bone grafts.

In another study, Inzana et al. tailored a composite scaffold using calcium phosphate and collagen for bone tissue regeneration [18]. Phosphoric acid at a concentration of 8.75 wt% was used as a binder that significantly improved the cellular viability. Tween 80 supplementation further enhanced the strength of the 3D printed scaffolds. Further, supplementation of the binder solution with 1–2 wt% collagen significantly enhanced the maximum flexural strength and cell viability. The pore size was in range from 20 to 50 μm that may significantly facilitate in-growth of the bone and

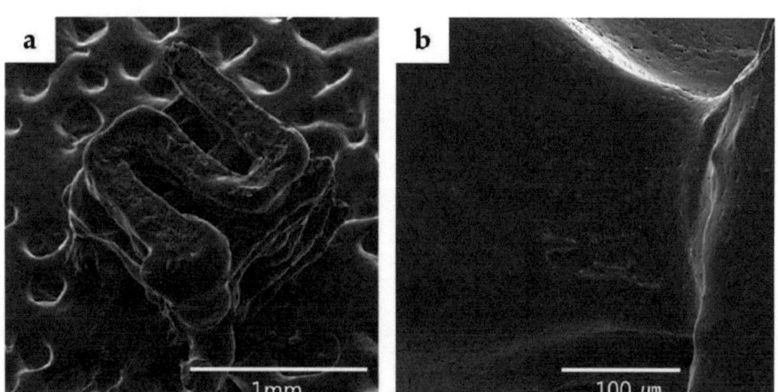

Figure 1.
SEM images of PCL/PLGA/β-TCP particulate bone grafts. (a) Well-defined PCL/PLGA/β-TCP particulate bone grafts were confirmed at a magnification of ×100; (b) rough surface of PCL/PLGA/β-TCP particulate hone grafts were observed at a magnification of ×800. Reprinted from Hwang et al. [17].

reestablishment of the marrow compartment. The surface was covered by plate like crystal growth which increased the surface area significantly that is ideal for adsorption of drugs and/or proteins. On implanting the 3D printed scaffolds into a critically sized murine femoral defect for 9 weeks, promising osteoconductive properties were noticed.

Kajave et al. (2021) developed a bioactive ink composed of Bioglass 45S5 (BG) and methacrylated collagen (CMA) for 3D printing of biomimetic constructs for bone tissue engineering [19]. The bioink resembled native bone tissue in the organic and inorganic composition. Superior stability with minimum swelling of the collagen based hydrogel was achieved due to homogeneous dispersion of BG particles within the collagen network. Excellent rheological property was confirmed by the betterment in the yield stress. Similarly, incorporation of the BG resulted in improvement in the percent recovery of 3D printed constructs. Additionally, improved bone bioactivity of 3D printed constructs in stimulated body fluid was advantageous. Osteogenic induction and differentiation by BG incorporated CMA (BG-CMA) constructs was associated with high cell viability and enhanced alkaline phosphatase activity and calcium deposition in human mesenchymal stem cells.

In another interesting study, Montalbano et al. fabricated a hybrid bioactive material suitable for 3D printing of scaffolds mimicking the natural composition and structure of healthy bone [20]. Initially mesoporous bioactive glass (BG) microspheres with 4% molar percentage of strontium were synthesized. Thereafter, Type I collagen and strontium-containing mesoporous BG were combined to obtain suspensions able to perform a sol–gel transition under physiological conditions. The fibrous nanostructures were homogeneously distributed embedding inorganic particles as evident from the field emission scanning electron microscopy (FESEM). Large calcium phosphate deposition was observed while release of strontium ions from the embedded BG was attributed to the high-water content of the composite. These features can cumulatively promote the osteogenic induction which is significant for bone tissue engineering. On soaking the composite scaffolds in simulated body fluid (SBF), hydroxyapatite (HA) crystals were uniformly distributed along the cross section of the sample that increased with time from 3rd to 7th day as evident from **Figure 2**.

In subsequent study Montalbano et al. reported composite biomimetics comprised of rod-like nano-hydroxyapatite particles embedded in a type I collagen matrix [21]. This composite was developed to mimic the bone composition. Initially a hydrothermal method using 0.2% ammonium-based dispersing agent (Darvan 821-A) was employed for the fabrication of the HA nanorods that were uniform-sized with length of 40–60 nm and a width of 20 nm. On suspending this material in a collagen solution in presence of Darvan 821-A, a uniform collagen/nano-HA suspension was obtained that was ideal for extrusion 3D printing. The mesh-like structures printed in a gelatine-supporting bath led to fabrication of 3D bone-like scaffolds.

2.2 Cartilage

One of the most prevalent tissue damages suffered by adults, children and adolescents is articular cartilage defects. In severe cases degenerative joint diseases may result due to exposure of bone terminals caused by progressive wear and tear of articular cartilage. However, low rate of tissue regeneration and self-repairing capacity poses a challenge for effective healing and restoration of the function. Several collagen based 3D scaffolds are being developed for inducing cartilage regeneration that is discussed in detail in this section. Recently, Lee et al. fabricated a highly biocompatible

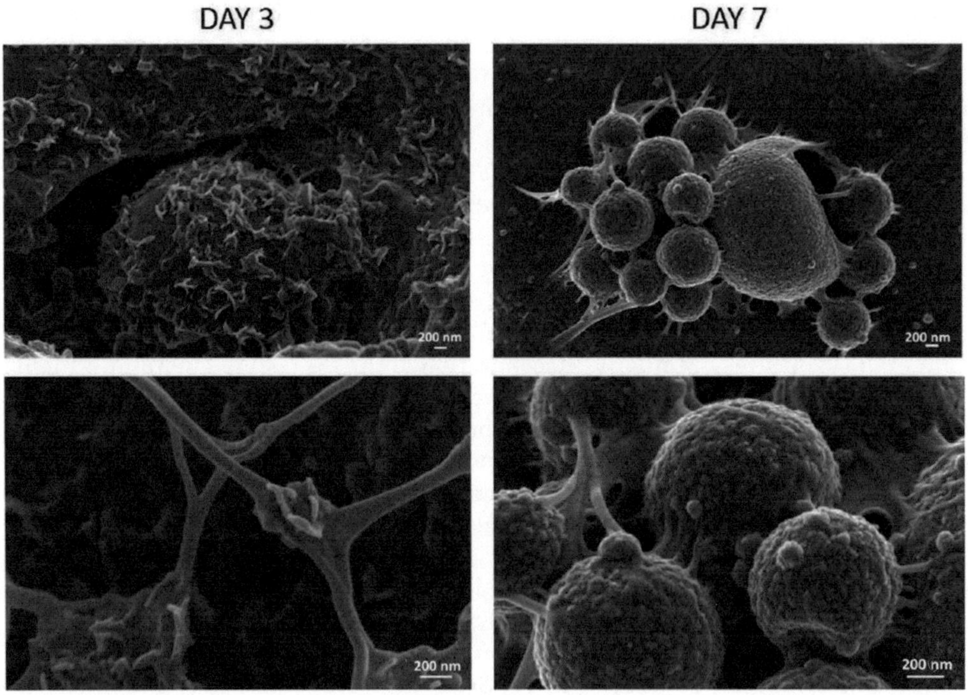

Figure 2.
Cross-sectional FESEM images showing HA crystal deposition on collagen/MBG_Sr4% samples after three and seven days of incubation in SBF at different magnifications. Reprinted from Montalbano et al. [20].

collagen/oligomeric proanthocyanidin/oxidized hyaluronic acid (C/OPC/OHA) composite scaffold with superior compressive strengths between 0.25–0.55 MPa [22]. The composite scaffolds were 3D printed using four types of needles, 25G red plastic, 22G blue plastic, 25G red metal, and 22G blue metal to achieve 20%, 25%, and 30% porosities when pressure of 25, 15, 125, and 100 kPa were applied, respectively as illustrated in **Figure 3**. Porous nature of the scaffolds is advantageous for promoting both angiogenesis and cartilage ossification. The minimum and maximum storage moduli of the hydrogel were approximately 2.6 kPa and 4.1 kPa, respectively. Interestingly, an increased degradation rate of the composites was 26.6%, 30%, and 30.7% for 0, 5, and 10 mg/mL of OHA, respectively after 49 days. Higher apatite deposition on the scaffold surface was evident on day 21 on immersion in simulated body fluid. Superior cell viability (up to 90%) was achieved when rat bone marrow mesenchymal stem cells (rBMSCs) were grown on the composite scaffolds. On implantation of the scaffolds into bone defects in skulls of the Sprague Dawley (SD) rat, angiogenesis and new bone formation was evident that indicated 3D collagen-based scaffolds could be used as potential candidates for articular cartilage repair.

Liu et al. developed a tri-layered scaffold employing extrusion-based multi-nozzle 3D printing technology where the bioink was comprised of 15% methacrylated gelatin (GelMA) hydrogel for cartilage on top layer, a combination of 20% GelMA and 3% nanohydroxyapatite (nHA) (20/3% GelMA/nHA) hydrogel for interfacial layer, and a 30/3% GelMA/nHA hydrogel for subchondral bone at bottom layer [23]. The composite was biodegradable with maximum degradation (61.4%) in 14 days. Interconnected microtubule-like structure of each layer with interconnected spherical pores with a

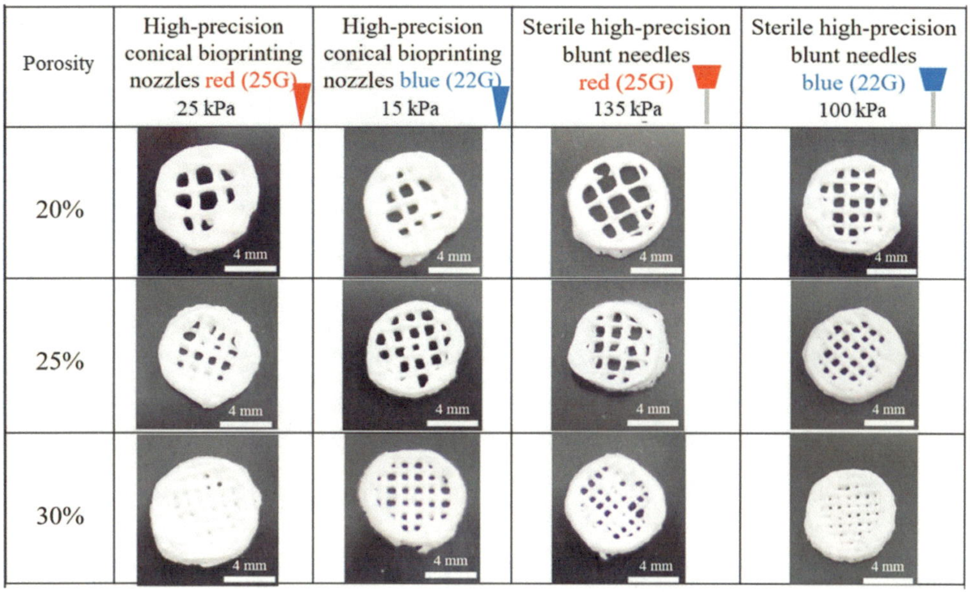

Figure 3.
Optimization of 3D bioprinting parameters for obtaining porosity at 20%, 25%, and 30% using different needle densities (25G red plastic and metal, 22G blue plastic and metal) and different pressures (25, 15, 135, and 100 kPa). Reprinted from Lee et al. [22].

size of about 300 μm was observed. The Young's modulus increased with the increase in GelMA concentration in the scaffold. The scaffolds were biocompatible with the bone marrow mesenchymal stem cells (BMSCs) while they exhibited effecting healing of rabbit osteochondral defect. Higher cartilage-specific extracellular matrix formation and collagen type II were observed on treatment with the tri-layered scaffolds. Further, effective new tissue formation and even integration with the surrounding tissues indicated their promises for repair of damages in subchondral bone by inducing cartilage regeneration.

In an interesting study, Rhee et al. fabricated 3D printing assisted soft tissue implants with high-density collagen hydrogels as illustrated in **Figure 4** [24]. External heating and collagen concentrations of 12.5, 15, and 17.5 mg/mL enhanced the shape fidelity. At the highest printable concentration, the modulus of printed gel was ~ 30 kPa. Cell viability within the tissue constructs was high and no notable decrease was observed even after 10 days of culturing. Higher infiltration of the fibochondrocytes cells throughout the collagen matrix was found by 10 days. Adherence of the cells on the outer surface of the nascent collagen fibers was prominent while very few cells colonized the spaces between the fibers.

2.3 Cardiac tissue (heart)

Cardio-vascular defects such as aortic valve disease (AVD) require high precision surgical procedure that include either mechanical or bioprosthetic valve replacement. Recently, tissue engineered heart valves (TEHV) have gained more attention that are effectively achieved by 3D bioprinting. Maxson et al. evaluated the recellularization potential of 3D-bioprinted scaffold and investigated its applicability as a heart valve implant [25]. Allogenic rat mesenchymal stem cells (rMSCs) with

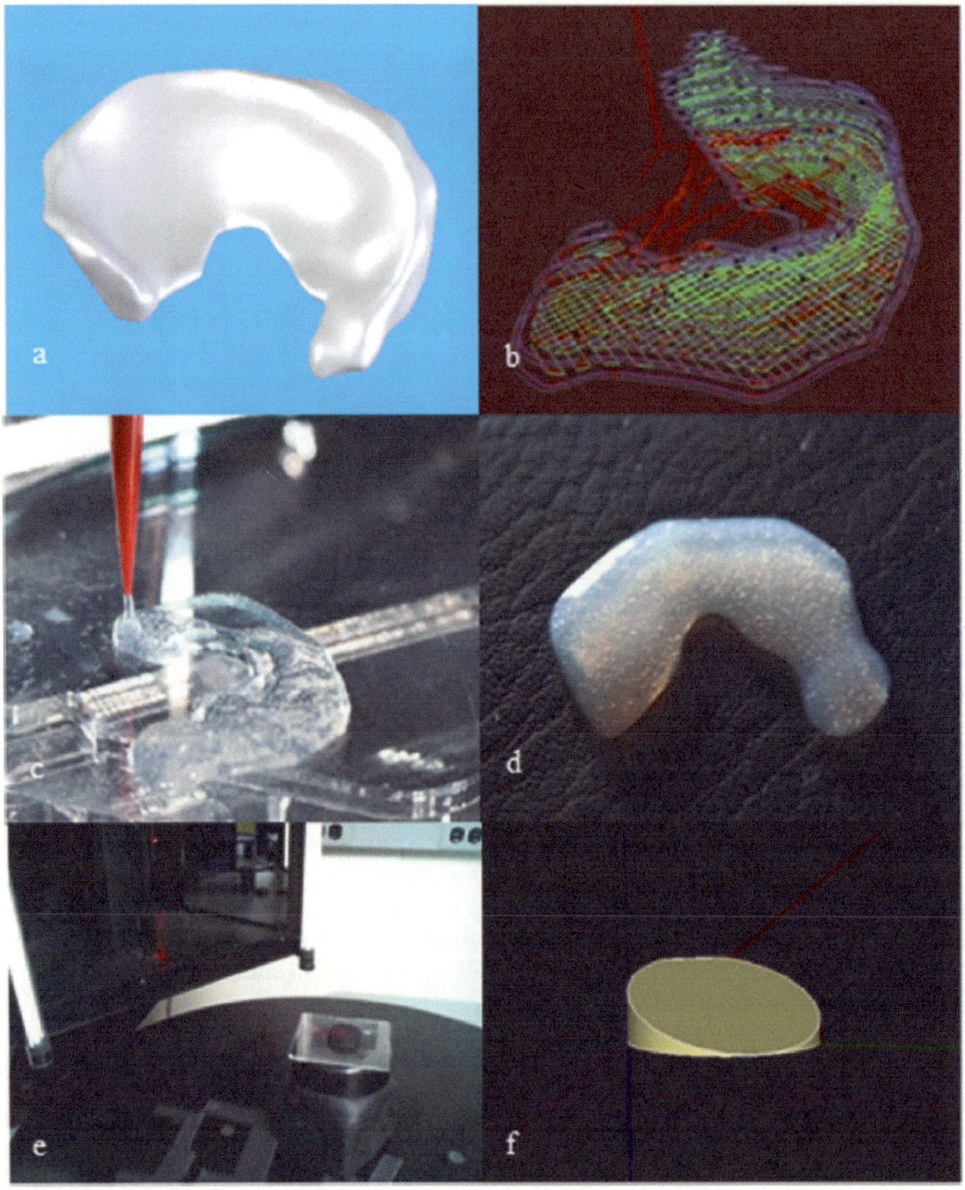

Figure 4.
Printing process of sheep meniscus, (a) CT scan of meniscus, (b) print path of meniscus deposition of collagen hydrogel during printing, (c) 3D printed meniscus. (d) Geometry assessment of constructs. (e) Constructs scanned using Cyberware 3D scanner. (f) Geometry of the test construct: Half-cylinder. Reprinted with permission from Rhee et al. [24]. Copyright © 2016 American Chemical Society.

green fluorescent protein (GFP) label were grown and mixed with Lifeink® 200 to obtain a homogenous bioink. Thereafter, a computer aided design (CAD) model for the implant disk scaffolds was prepared wherein the dimensions of the scaffold facilitated easy implantation and mounting in order to avoid migration and folding. Neovascularization was observed after 4 weeks with integration of host tissues with the bioink explants. Moreover after 8 weeks, minimal difference between the two layers was observed; however, the structural integrity of the extracellular matrix (ECM) was maintained. Furthermore, Mason's trichome revealed fibrosis on the cutaneous side of the explant whereas CD3 and CD163 biomarkers demonstrated chronic inflammation as well as ECM remodeling whose expressions were decreased with subsequent increase in incubation period. CD163 displayed a steady reduction in expression from week 1 to week 8, respectively. On the other hand, CD31 biomarker expression was considerably increased within the same time period due to endothelialization and angiogenesis. The vimentin (a major intermediate filament of smooth muscle cells) concentration of surrounding tissues was also increased with improvement in elastin concentration. This was attributed to the infiltration of the Bioink by interstitial-like cells. In addition, the ultimate tensile strength (UTS) was decreased from 0.344 ± 0.120 MPa in the second week to 0.169 ± 0.077 MPa in the fourth week while it was increased to 0.275 ± 0.166 MPa in the eighth week. Likewise, the tensile modulus was also reduced from 1.186 ± 0.872 MPa in the second week to 0.548 ± 0.341 MPa in the fourth week followed by an increase to 1.425 ± 0.620 MPa in the eighth week. Elastin concentration was significantly increased in the fourth week. Post eight weeks of implantation, expression of CD31 biomarker continued to decrease while CD163 expression increased in week 12 which was attributed to M2 macrophage infiltration. Additionally, the bioink explant was encapsulated by the fibrotic tissue within week 12 while UTS was further increased within this time period. Enhanced levels of both vimentin and elastin indicated strengthening of the extracellular matrix in the bioprinted scaffold due to active collagen deposition. Hence, collagen-based bioink application was demonstrated to be efficient for formation of heart valves.

In another study, Lee et al. also demonstrated 3D bioprinting of collagen for human heart engineering [12]. Herein, 3D bioprinting was carried out using a second generation of the free form reversible embedding of suspended hydrogels (FRESH v2.0) that provides support for printing and then subsequently melts away at 37°C. Moreover, uniform gelatin microparticles with spherical morphology (with diameter ~ 25 μm) reduced polydispersity. An optimal balance between the resolution of individual strand and strand-to-strand adhesion was further maintained using a 50 mM N-2-hydroxyethylpiperazine-N′-2-ethanesulfonic acid (HEPES) buffered bath with pH 7.4 which in turn facilitated multiple bioink printing. A linear small coronary artery-scale tube was then fabricated using collagen type I perfusion system with an inner diameter and wall thickness of 1.4 mm and 300 μm, respectively. Thereafter, C2C12 cells were perfused in the tube that displayed viability along with active remodeling of the gel after five days. Further, cellular infiltration was also analyzed using fabrication of collagen disks with a thickness of 5 mm and a diameter of 10 mm wherein excessive cellular infiltration as well as collagen remodeling was observed post three days of implantation in the printed collagen as compared to solid-cast collagen. Moreover, fibronectin and vascular endothelial growth factor (VEGF) were incorporated into the bioink for enhanced vascularization. An extensive vascular network was observed in the printed collagen disk with red blood cells and CD31-positive vessels having a diameter range of 8–50 μm. Thereafter, collagen bioink was used along with human stem cell-derived cardiomyocytes to FRESH print a left ventricle model wherein around 96% post-printing cell viability was achieved through rapid collagen neutralization. A dense layer of interconnected and striated human embryonic stem cell-cardiomyocytes (hESC-CMs) was obtained after seven days of culturing. A baseline spontaneous ventricle beat rate of around 0.5 Hz was captured that was paced at 1 and 2 Hz using field stimulation. Furthermore, the mechanical integrity of the constructs was demonstrated using a 28 mm tri-leaflet heart valve that was robust enough to withstand air pressure. In addition, a neonatal-scale human heart was also printed using collagen bioink that highlighted the potential of FRESH v2.0 printing technique for fabrication of advanced tissue scaffolds for other organ systems as well.

Collagen-based bio-ink was also demonstrated to be an effective tool for direct 3D printing of human induced pluripotent stem cells (hiPSC)-cardiomyocytes that could then be utilized for cardiac tissue engineering [26]. Cardiomyocytes were differentiated in a 2D monolayer followed by CHIR99021-treatment mediated cell expansion and regular passing. Later on, a rat collagen-I based bioink was used for the encapsulation of cells followed by printing in a support bath composed of complex coacervate gelatin/gum arabic microparticles. The bioink was then gelated at 37°C and cultivated under free-floating conditions for a time period of thirty days. Ring-shaped cardiac tissues were printed with 5 × 5 × 1 mm dimension wherein the initial contractions were seen post three days of culturing. Striated sarcomeres were demonstrated with significant responsiveness toward pharmacological stimulations. Therefore, this study demonstrated potential of cardiac tissue engineering with enhanced properties and functions through 3D-bioprinting.

2.4 Nerve

Scaffolds rationally fabricated employing 3D bioprinting could help in the treatment of spinal cord injury (SCI) by nerve tissue engineering. In a study by Jiang et al., Collagen/silk fibroin scaffold was 3D bioprinted and combined with neural stem cells (NSCs) to promote nerve regeneration [27]. A collagen/silk fibroin ratio of 4:2 was used for scaffold preparation using a 3D-bioprinter with a nozzle diameter of 210 μm, printing speed of 9 mm, extrusion speed of 2-mm/min, 0.1 mm thickness and a platform temperature of −20°C. Characterization of the 3D bioprinted scaffolds in rats revealed complete degradation of the composite scaffold after 4 weeks of implantation. Furthermore, the scaffold had considerable ductility as well as compression resistance with a compressive elastic modulus of 60.05 ± 5.12 kPa. Fourier transform infrared (FTIR) spectroscopy results then revealed presence of absorption peaks at 3445.7, 2932.46, 1640.58, and 1376.45 cm^{-1} that corresponded with -OH or -NH peak, methyl or C-H stretching vibrations of methylene group, C=O or C=C stretching vibrations, and saturated C-H bending vibration, respectively. Hence, these functional groups suggested presence of suitable lipid- and water-soluble bonds in the 3D bioprinted scaffold that may facilitate adhesion and growth of nerve cells. Moreover, significant biocompatibility between the scaffold and NSCs were attained with evenly distributed micropores and pore connections in the scaffold as observed in scanning electron microscopy (SEM) images. Fusiform-shaped cells grew in the scaffold pores, while some cells grew densely on the scaffold surface with extended pseudopods facilitating cell adhesion, growth as well as provided a carrier and channel for regeneration of the nerve fibers. Hence, a conducive microenvironment for NSC adhesion, growth and differentiation was provided by the 3D-bioprinted scaffold. Furthermore, 3-(4,5-dimethylthiazol-2-yl)-2,5-diphenyl tetrazolium bromide (MTT) assay also demonstrated successful seeding and proliferation of the NSCs on the scaffold. Thereafter, behavioral changes at the spinal cord injury site were investigated after implantation of the scaffold. The Basso-Beattie-Bresnahan (BBB) open-field locomotor score of the group implanted with 3D-collagen/silk fibroin scaffolds and NSCs was higher as compared to the control after 8 weeks of surgery. In addition, motor function recovery was better in groups having the scaffold and

NSCs. Similarly, electrophysiological studies revealed prominent recovery in groups having 3D bioprinted scaffold along with NSCs as compared to control groups. Left hind limb amplitude was significantly higher in scaffold group when compared with control after 1 month of surgery. In addition, magnetic resonance imaging (MRI) and diffusion tensor imaging revealed improved filling of the injury cavity, enhanced spinal cord continuity, increased regenerative axons as well as reduced glial scarring in groups implanted with the scaffold and NSCs.

In another study, Li and Gao fabricated 3D microtubular collagen scaffolds and investigated its potential in peripheral nerve repair [28]. Melt spinning or 3D printing using poly-lactic acid (PLA) was carried out to obtain fibrous template material with a diameter range of 50–100 μm that was then utilized for fabrication of collagen scaffolds. Microtubules were prepared by parallel stacking of melt spun PLA fibers followed by polymerization of the collagen whereas PLA fibers with a diameter of 200 μm and 100 μm interspacing was fused and deposited using 3D printing. The thickness of inner ranged from 10 to 20 μm while the exterior wall formed a shell with a thickness of about 70 μm. Furthermore, cell adhesion ability of adrenal phaeochromocytoma (PC-12) and D62PT Schwann cells was evaluated wherein the cells firmly attached to native as well as chloroform-exposed Matrigel films. Two crosslinkers namely, 0.3% genipin and 0.3% glutaraldehyde were used that decreased swelling as well as enzymatic degradation of the Matrigel. Untreated gels demonstrated retention of 34.5% of total mass after 24 h incubation with 0.05% collagenase, whereas genipin and glutaraldehyde treated gels showed total mass retention of 96.7% and 99.3%, respectively. PC-12 and D62PT Schwann cells further showed well adherence and confluent growth onto microtubule scaffolds after 10 and 4–5 days of culturing, respectively. Moreover, a strong alignment of cells as well as formation of channels was seen in Schwann cells while primary chick dorsal root ganglia displayed neurite growth along the major axis of the microtubes.

Likewise, Yoo et al. reported fabrication of elastic nerve guidance conduits (NGCs) using poly(lactide-*co*-caprolactone) (PLCL) along with a 3D printed collagen hydrogel [29]. A dense acidified collagen solution with a viscosity of 1.3×10^5 mPa s was used as the bio-ink to print onto the electrospun PLCL membrane that had an optimal porosity of 2.7 ± 0.6 μm which allowed nutrient and oxygen exchange only. The acidified collagen hydrogel was then neutralized using ammonia vapor which prevented crumbling of the hydrogel. Thereafter, the NGCs were shaped into tubes and implanted in the rat sciatic nerve model. SEM images of the longitudinal cross-section of the NGCs demonstrated consistent gel deposition wherein the pore size was reduced by extraction of nano-sized fibers which in turn, prevented cell penetration into the NGCs. Moreover, a conduit fill ratio of 72 ± 2% was observed based on the hydrated cross-sectional images. Furthermore, the biocompatibility of the prepared composite was evaluated using PC12 cell culturing on the PLCL membrane with the 3D printed collagen hydrogel. After 1 week of PC12 cell culturing, a neuron-like elongated differentiation was observed in cells that were grown on the PLCL membrane having 3D printed collagen hydrogel whereas no such differentiation was observed in cells cultured on native PLCL membrane. In addition, no significant differences in the weight percentage of different animal groups were observed as well as no signs of infection, delayed wound healing, or auto-mutilation was observed throughout the experiment. The ankle contracture angles of 3D printing group after 12 weeks of nerve reconstruction was 89.68 ± 2.37% as compared to 93.52 ± 3.17% and 83.86 ± 4.64% for the autograft and bulk collagen groups, respectively. Likewise, the active ankle angle at terminal stance (ATS) was improved in 3D printing and autograft groups after twelve weeks of nerve reconstruction with angle values of as compared to 24.02 ± 1.26° and 19.65 ± 4.78°, respectively as compared to 11.35 ± 2.91° in the case of bulk group. Hence, it was proved that 3D printed collagen hydrogel facilitated motor regeneration using NGCs. Furthermore, a comparable tetanic force of tibialis anterior (TA) muscles was observed in the 3D printing and autograft groups after twelve weeks while the bulk group displayed a lower tetanic force. The nerve regeneration through NGCs was observed after twelve weeks of surgery with linear guidance of the 3D printed collagen hydrogel from the proximal to distal ends along with an organized pattern of the regenerated axons. Moreover, the myelinated axon counts as well as thickness of myelin in the 3D printing group was higher than the bulk group. Additionally, the myelin fiber area and nerve fiber density of 3D printing group were 53,134 ± 5893 μm^2 and 11,206 ± 1980 n mm^{-2}, respectively.

Lee et al. also demonstrated bio-printing of collagen and VEGF-releasing fibrin gel scaffolds and investigated its potential in artificial neural tissue construction [30]. Murine neural stem cells (NSCs) were cultured in Dulbecco's modified Eagle's medium (DMEM) and further used for cell printing. Type I collagen was then prepared and 1.16 mg/mL of the collagen scaffold was used for 3D bio-printing of C17.2 cell-scaffold complex. An average of 56 ± 9 cells/droplet was obtained with a cell viability of 93.23 ± 3.77% which was similar to that of manually-plated cells. Moreover, a collagen scaffold concentration of 1.74 mg/mL demonstrated highly dense and proliferating cells with a viability of 96.72 ± 3.58% after 3 days of culturing. Furthermore, the combinatorial effect of collagen scaffold and VEGF-containing fibrin gel on C17.2 cells was investigated wherein, the cell morphology altered after two days of culturing with active proliferation and formation of clusters. In addition, the cells located near the fibrin gel border gradually migrated toward the VEGF-containing fibrin gel and continued differentiation. After three days of culturing, the total migration distance was 102.4 ± 76.1 μm. Hence, proper cell proliferation and migration was displayed using the two scaffolds which highlighted the potential of 3D bioprinting in artificial tissue construction.

Likewise, axon regeneration was ameliorated by Sun et al. using 3D printed collagen/chitosan scaffolds [31]. A 3D bioprinter was used for fabrication of the scaffold that had an interconnected porous structure with a porosity of 83.5% as observed in SEM images. The pore size of the scaffold ranged from 60 to 200 μm. Hence, significant space was obtained by the cells for growth and adherence. The compressive modulus of 3D collagen/chitosan scaffold was 3.82 ± 0.25 MPa along with enhanced compressive strength of 345.20 ± 29.60 KPa. The cytocompatibility of 3D printed scaffolds was similar to that of scaffolds prepared using freeze drying technology. Interestingly, the persistent locomotion recovery as well as significant increase in blood brain barrier (BBB) scores was observed after implantation of the 3D printed collagen/chitosan scaffolds in rats with spinal cord injury (SCI). Moreover, the magnetic resonance and diffusion tensor imaging results revealed a significant signal increase at the epicenter of the spinal cord lesion in rats implanted with 3D printed collagen/chitosan scaffold. Post eight weeks of SCI surgery, the axonal regeneration was demonstrated wherein 3D collagen/chitosan implantations resulted in amplitude and latency improvement. Further confirmation of axonal regeneration was carried out using anterograde biotin dextran amine (BDA) labeling wherein BDA-positive fibers were observed in 3D collagen/chitosan implantations. Hematoxylin and eosin (HE) staining also demonstrated linear ordered structure of the spinal cord after eight weeks with no obvious cavity observed in 3D printed collagen/chitosan implanted group whereas visible cavities and disordered structures were observed in injury groups. Hence, 3D printed scaffolds were demonstrated to be effective in axon regeneration and amelioration of spinal cord injury.

In a similar study, Chen et al. constructed collagen/heparin sulfate based scaffolds using 3D bioprinting and evaluated its action in functional SCI recovery in rats [13]. The scaffold was prepared using a 3D bioprinter that had a cylindrical morphology with a uniform and regular internal structure along with high porosity as observed in SEM images. The compressive modulus of 3D printed collagen/heparin sulfate was 3.46 ± 0.278 MPa which was higher as compared to scaffolds prepared using freeze drying technology. Likewise, enhanced compressive strength of 308.9 ± 28.65 KPa was observed in 3D printed scaffold. Furthermore, release profile of basic fibroblast growth factor (bFGF) from 3D printed scaffold was also evaluated wherein scaffolds prepared using freeze drying method demonstrated an initial burst of 54.89% of bFGF was released in the first day after which a slow release behavior was observed for longer time period. However, a steady bFGF release behavior was observed in case of 3D printed scaffolds for twenty days. Thereafter, the biocompatibility of scaffolds was analyzed using NSCs which proliferated inside the pore followed by spreading on the wall of the scaffolds. In addition, MTT assay revealed no significant difference in cell growth on different scaffolds thus highlighting the cytocompatibility of the 3D printed collagen/heparin sulfate scaffolds. Implantation of the 3D printed scaffolds further demonstrated significant recovery of locomotor functions in rats after two months with amelioration of the SCI as well as enhanced number of neurofilament positive cells.

3. Conclusions and future perspectives

Advances in the field of nanomedicine have enabled exploration of novel biomaterials for tissue engineering. Among various biopolymers such as, chitosan, alginate, silk fibrion, collagen is considered as most attractive due to its biocompatibility and biodegradability. However, high temperature and extreme conditions during fabrication and bioprinting results in low stability of the collagen molecules. Hence, ideal porous scaffolds should involve combination of type I collagen and hydroxyapatite particles by freeze-drying. It is essential to have tuneable pore dimensions for superior ingrowth of cells and blood vessels. More complex microarchitectures of the collagen based scaffolds with specific rheological properties such as shear thinning, yield stress and fast shear recovery can be obtained using extrusion-based 3D printing [33].

Various biologically synthesized nanoparticles like silver, gold, copper, platinum, palladium and others can be supplemented in the scaffolds resisting post-surgical microbial infections [34–37]. Biofilm associated infections are most challenging to treat and are highly responsible for implant failure. Hence, coating of implants with antimicrobial nanoparticles impregnated collagen can be an effective strategy to increase the shelf life of the implants [38, 39]. Also drug functionalized nanoparticles can be embedded in the collagen matrix to ensure sustained release and rapid healing of the injured tissues.

Multiple approaches and integration of medical biology and material science will certainly help to revolutionize regenerative medicine by rational tissue engineering. In view of the background collagen based 3D printed scaffolds hold tremendous potential as candidate nanotherapeutics.

Acknowledgements

Dr. Sougata Ghosh acknowledges Kasetsart University, Bangkok, Thailand for Post Doctoral Fellowship and funding under Reinventing University Program (Ref. No. 6501.0207/10870 dated 9th November, 2021).

Conflict of interest

The authors declare no conflict of interest.

Author details

Sougata Ghosh[1,2]*, Bishwarup Sarkar[3], Ratnakar Mishra[4], Nanasaheb Thorat[5] and Sirikanjana Thongmee[1]

1 Faculty of Science, Department of Physics, Kasetsart University, Bangkok, Thailand

2 Department of Microbiology, School of Science, RK University, Rajkot, Gujarat, India

3 College of Science, Northeastern University, Boston, MA, USA

4 Cambridge Centre for Brain Repair and MRC Mitochondrial Biology Unit, Department of Clinical Neurosciences, University of Cambridge, Cambridge, UK

5 Nuffield Department of Women's and Reproductive Health, Division of Medical Sciences, John Radcliffe Hospital, University of Oxford, Oxford, UK

*Address all correspondence to: ghoshsibb@gmail.com

References

[1] O'Brien FJ. Biomaterials & scaffolds for tissue engineering. Materials Today. 2011;**14**:88-95. DOI: 10.1016/S1369-7021(11)70058-X

[2] Ghosh S, Mostafavi E, Thorat N, Webster TJ. Nanobiomaterials for three-dimensional bioprinting. In: Liu H, Shokuhfar T, Ghosh S, editors. Nanotechnology in Medicine and Biology. Amsterdam, Netherlands: Elsevier; 2021. pp. 1-24. DOI: 10.1016/B978-0-12-819469-0.00003-4

[3] Kohane DS, Langer R. Polymeric biomaterials in tissue engineering. Pediatric Research. 2008;**63**:487-491. DOI: 10.1203/01.pdr.0000305937.26105.e7

[4] Nguyen QT, Hwang Y, Chen AC, Varghese S, Sah RL. Cartilage-like mechanical properties of poly (ethylene glycol)-diacrylate hydrogels. Biomaterials. 2012;**33**:6682-6690. DOI: 10.1016/j.biomaterials.2012.06.005

[5] Ghosh S, Webster TJ. Metallic nanoscaffolds as osteogenic promoters: Advances, challenges and scope. Metals. 2021a;**11**:1356. DOI: 10.3390/met11091356

[6] Ghosh S, Webster TJ. Mesoporous silica based nanostructures for bone tissue regeneration. Frontiers in Materials. 2021b;**8**:692309. DOI: 10.3389/fmats.2021.692309

[7] Kolk A, Handschel J, Drescher W, Rothamel D, Kloss F, Blessmann M, et al. Current trends and future perspectives of bone substitute materials—From space holders to innovative biomaterials. Journal of Cranio-Maxillo-Facial Surgery. 2012;**40**:706-718. DOI: 10.1016/j.jcms.2012.01.002

[8] Greenberg SE, VanHouten J, Lakomkin N, Ehrenfeld J, Jahangir AA, Boyce RH, et al. Does admission to medicine or orthopaedics impact a geriatric hip Patient's hospital length of stay? Journal of Orthopaedic Trauma. 2016;**30**:95-99. DOI: 10.1097/BOT.0000000000000440

[9] Pathria MN, Chung CB, Resnick DL. Acute and stress-related injuries of bone and cartilage: Pertinent anatomy, basic biomechanics, and imaging perspective. Radiology. 2016;**280**:21-38. DOI: 10.1148/radiol.16142305

[10] Wong C-C, Chen C-H, Chiu L-H, Tsuang Y-H, Bai M-Y, Chung R-J, et al. Facilitating in vivo articular cartilage repair by tissue-engineered cartilage grafts produced from auricular chondrocytes. The American Journal of Sports Medicine. 2018;**46**:713-727. DOI: 10.1177/0363546517741306

[11] Basad E, Wissing FR, Fehrenbach P, Rickert M, Steinmeyer J, Ishaque B. Matrix-induced autologous chondrocyte implantation (MACI) in the knee: Clinical outcomes and challenges. Knee Surgery, Sports Traumatology, Arthroscopy. 2015;**23**:3729-3735. DOI: 10.1007/s00167-014-3295-8

[12] Lee AR, Hudson AR, Shiwarski DJ, Tashman JW, Hinton TJ, Yerneni S, et al. 3D bioprinting of collagen to rebuild components of the human heart. Science. 2019;**365**(6452):482-487. DOI: 10.1126/science.aav9051

[13] Chen C, Zhao ML, Zhang RK, Lu G, Zhao CY, Fu F, et al. Collagen/heparin sulfate scaffolds fabricated by a 3D bioprinter improved mechanical properties and neurological function after spinal cord injury in rats. Journal of

Biomedical Materials Research. Part A. 2017;**105**(5):1324-1332. DOI: 10.1002/jbm.a.36011

[14] Yamazaki CM, Kadoya Y, Hozumi K, Okano-Kosugi H, Asada S, Kitagawa K, et al. A collagen-mimetic triple helical supramolecule that evokes integrin-dependent cell responses. Biomaterials. 2010;**31**:1925-1934. DOI: 10.1016/j.biomaterials.2009.10.014

[15] Chevallay B, Herbage D. Collagen-based biomaterials as 3D scaffold for cell cultures: Applications for tissue engineering and gene therapy. Medical & Biological Engineering & Computing. 2000;**38**:211-218. DOI: 10.1007/BF02344779

[16] Wolf K, Alexander S, Schacht V, Coussens LM, von Andrian UH, van Rheenen J, et al. Collagen-based cell migration models in vitro and in vivo. Seminars in Cell & Developmental Biology. 2009;**20**:931-941. DOI: 10.1016/j.semcdb.2009.08.005

[17] Hwang KS, Choi JW, Kim JH, Chung HY, Jin S, Shim JH, et al. Comparative efficacies of collagen-based 3D printed PCL/PLGA/β-TCP composite block bone grafts and biphasic calcium phosphate bone substitute for bone regeneration. Materials. 2017;**10**:421. DOI: 10.3390/ma10040421

[18] Inzana JA, Olvera D, Fuller SM, Kelly JP, Graeve OA, Schwarz EM, et al. 3D printing of composite calcium phosphate and collagen scaffolds for bone regeneration. Biomaterials. 2014;**35**:4026-4034. DOI: 10.1016/j.biomaterials.2014.01.064

[19] Kajave NS, Schmitt T, Nguyen T-U, Gaharwar AK, Kishore V. Bioglass incorporated methacrylated collagen bioactive ink for 3D printing of bone tissue. Biomedical Materials. 2021;**16**:035003. DOI: 10.1088/1748-605X/abc744

[20] Montalbano G, Fiorilli S, Caneschi A, Vitale-Brovarone C. Type I collagen and strontium-containing mesoporous glass particles as hybrid material for 3D printing of bone-like materials. Materials. 2018;**11**:700. DOI: 10.3390/ma11050700

[21] Montalbano G, Molino G, Fiorilli S, Vitale-Brovarone C. Synthesis and incorporation of rod-like nano-hydroxyapatite into type I collagen matrix: A hybrid formulation for 3D printing of bone scaffolds. Journal of the European Ceramic Society. 2020;**40**:3689-3697. DOI: 10.1016/j.jeurceramsoc.2020.02.018

[22] Lee C-F, Hsu Y-H, Lin Y-C, Nguyen T-T, Chen H-W, Nabilla SC, et al. 3D printing of collagen/oligomeric proanthocyanidin/oxidized hyaluronic acid composite scaffolds for articular cartilage repair. Polymers. 2021;**13**:3123. DOI: 10.3390/polym13183123

[23] Liu J, Li L, Suo H, Yan M, Yin J, Fu J. 3D printing of biomimetic multi-layered GelMA/nHA scaffold for osteochondral defect repair. Materials and Design. 2019;**171**:107708. DOI: 10.1016/j.matdes.2019.107708

[24] Rhee S, Puetzer JL, Mason BN, Reinhart-King CA, Bonassar LJ. 3D bioprinting of spatially heterogeneous collagen constructs for cartilage tissue engineering. ACS Biomaterials Science & Engineering. 2016;**2**:1800-1805. DOI: 10.1021/acsbiomaterials.6b00288

[25] Maxson EL, Young MD, Noble C, Go JL, Heidari B, Khorramirouz R, et al. In vivo remodeling of a 3D-bioprinted tissue engineered heart valve scaffold. Bioprinting. 2019;**16**:e00059. DOI: 10.1016/j.bprint.2019.e00059

[26] Esser TU, Engel FB. Direct 3D printing of hiPSC-cardiomyocytes in collagen-based bioinks. European Heart Journal. 2021;**42**(Supplement_1):3236. DOI: 10.1093/eurheartj/ehab724.3236

[27] Jiang JP, Liu XY, Zhao F, Zhu X, Li XY, Niu XG, et al. Three-dimensional bioprinting collagen/silk fibroin scaffold combined with neural stem cells promotes nerve regeneration after spinal cord injury. Neural Regeneration Research. 2020;**15**(5):959-968. DOI: 10.4103/1673-5374.268974

[28] Li J, Gao W. Fabrication and characterization of 3D microtubular collagen scaffolds for peripheral nerve repair. Journal of Biomaterials Applications. 2018;**33**(4):541-552. DOI: 10.1177/0885328218804338

[29] Yoo J, Park JH, Kwon YW, Chung JJ, Choi IC, Nam JJ, et al. Augmented peripheral nerve regeneration through elastic nerve guidance conduits prepared using a porous PLCL membrane with a 3D printed collagen hydrogel. Biomaterials Science. 2020;**8**:6261-6271. DOI: 10.1039/D0BM00847H

[30] Lee YB, Polio S, Lee W, Dai G, Menon L, Carroll RS, et al. Bio-printing of collagen and VEGF-releasing fibrin gel scaffolds for neural stem cell culture. Experimental Neurology. 2010;**223**(2):645-652. DOI: 10.1016/j.expneurol.2010.02.014

[31] Sun Y, Yang C, Zhu X, Wang JJ, Liu XY, Yang XP, et al. 3D printing collagen/chitosan scaffold ameliorated axon regeneration and neurological recovery after spinal cord injury. Journal of Biomedial Materials Research Part A. 2019;**107**(9):1898-1908. DOI: 10.1002/jbm.a.36675

[32] Osidak EO, Kozhukhov VI, Osidak MS, Domogatsky SP. Collagen as bioink for bioprinting: A comprehensive review. International Journal of Bioprinting. 2020;**6**(3):270. DOI: 10.18063/ijb.v6i3.270

[33] Ghosh S, Sanghavi S, Sancheti P. Metallic biomaterial for bone support and replacement. In: Balakrishnan P, Sreekala MS, Thomas S, editors. Fundamental Biomaterials: Metals. Vol 2. United Kingdom: Woodhead Publishing Series in Biomaterials. Woodhead Publishing; 2018. pp. 139-165. DOI: 10.1016/B978-0-08-102205-4.00006-4

[34] Ghosh S, Patil S, Chopade NB, Luikham S, Kitture R, Gurav DD, et al. *Gnidia glauca* leaf and stem extract mediated synthesis of gold nanocatalysts with free radical scavenging potential. Journal of Nanomedicine & Nanotechnology. 2016a;7:358. DOI: 10.4172/2157-7439.1000358

[35] Ghosh S, Harke AN, Chacko MJ, Gurav SP, Joshi KA, Dhepe A, et al. *Gloriosa superba* mediated synthesis of silver and gold nanoparticles for anticancer applications. Journal of Nanomedicine & Nanotechnology. 2016b;7:4. DOI: 10.4172/2157-7439.1000390

[36] Ghosh S, Chacko MJ, Harke AN, Gurav SP, Joshi KA, Dhepe A, et al. *Barleria prionitis* leaf mediated synthesis of silver and gold nanocatalysts. Journal of Nanomedicine & Nanotechnology. 2016c;7:4. DOI: 10.4172/2157-7439.1000394

[37] Ghosh S, Gurav SP, Harke AN, Chacko MJ, Joshi KA, Dhepe A, et al. *Dioscorea oppositifolia* mediated synthesis of gold and silver nanoparticles with catalytic activity. Journal of Nanomedicine & Nanotechnology. 2016d;7:5. DOI: 10.4172/2157-7439.1000398

[38] Bloch K, Pardesi K, Satriano C, Ghosh S. Bacteriogenic platinum nanoparticles for application in nanomedicine. Frontiers in Chemistry. 2021;**9**:624344. DOI: 10.3389/fchem.2021.624344

[39] Ranpariya B, Salunke G, Karmakar S, Babiya K, Sutar S, Kadoo N, et al. Antimicrobial synergy of silver-platinum nanohybrids with antibiotics. Frontiers in Microbiology. 2021;**11**:610968. DOI: 10.3389/fmicb.2020.610968

Chapter 7

Mechanical Methods of Producing Biomaterials with Aligned Collagen Fibrils

Shunji Yunoki, Eiji Kondo and Kazunori Yasuda

Abstract

Collagen has been used in various therapeutic medical devices, such as artificial dermis, bone, and cartilage, wherein the effectiveness of collagen mainly depends on its biological features of biocompatibility, biodegradability, bioresorbability, cell affinity, and weak antigenicity. Collagen is the main structural protein in the human body and is responsible for the mechanical properties of tissues and organs. The fundamental structural component of tendon tissue is uniaxially aligned collagen fibrils that run parallel to the geometrical axis. Thus, the fabrication of artificial tendons is an excellent example of developing biomaterials using collagen as a structural backbone. Previous attempts to construct aligned fibril-based biomaterials involved electrospinning, freeze drying, using a strong magnetic field, and mechanical methods, including shearing and tension during wet extrusion. Among these, mechanical methods have been extensively studied owing to their simplicity and effectiveness suitable for mass production. However, few review articles have focused on these mechanical methods. Thus, this article reviews the mechanical methods for creating biomaterials from aligned collagen fibril while discussing the other fabrication methods in brief.

Keywords: tendon, collagen, fibril, alignment, shearing

1. Introduction

Since the research and development of collagen-based artificial dermis began in the 1980s [1, 2], many biomaterials using collagen as the base have been developed and clinically applied [3, 4]. Currently, many advanced collagen-based biomaterials have been developed for cellular or acellular tissue engineering and cell therapies [5, 6], and collagen remains one of the most essential biomaterials. Collagen is useful as a base material for therapeutic biomaterials due to its excellent biochemical properties (biocompatibility, biodegradability, and bioabsorbability) [3, 4] and cell affinity [5]. These properties enable the resultant biomaterials to be decomposed through biological activity, absorbed and metabolized at the damaged sites, and eventually be replaced with normal tissues. The effectiveness of collagen in such biomaterials primarily depends on the abovementioned biological features as well as its weak antigenicity. Its excellent moldability and low cost have further facilitated the development of sheet-shaped artificial dermis [7], porous artificial bones [8], and hydrogel-based artificial cartilages [9].

However, the mechanical properties of such collagen-based biomaterials and artificial tissues are significantly inferior to those of living tissues. Collagen is the main

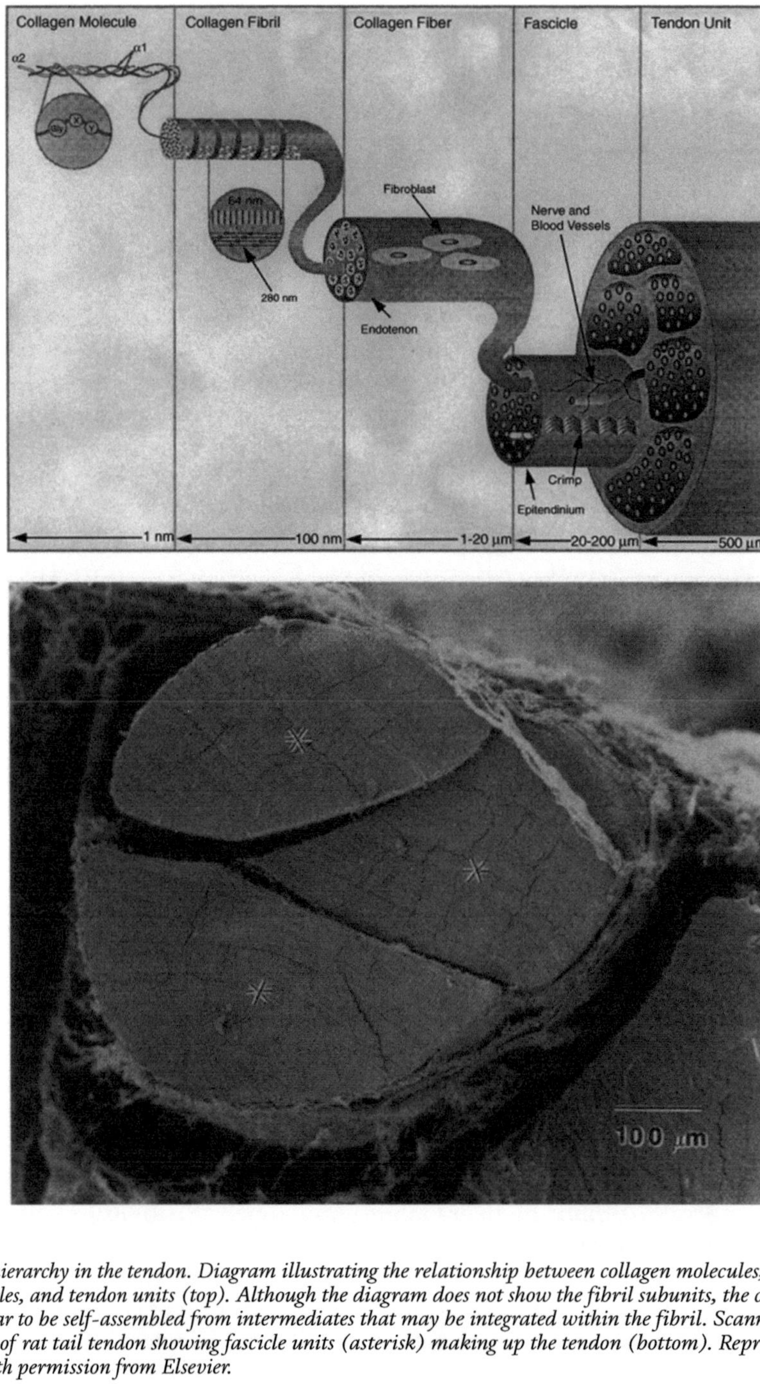

Figure 1.
Structural hierarchy in the tendon. Diagram illustrating the relationship between collagen molecules, fibrils, fibers, fascicles, and tendon units (top). Although the diagram does not show the fibril subunits, the collagen fibrils appear to be self-assembled from intermediates that may be integrated within the fibril. Scanning electron micrograph of rat tail tendon showing fascicle units (asterisk) making up the tendon (bottom). Reproduced from Ref. [11] with permission from Elsevier.

structural protein in the human body and is responsible for the mechanical features of tissues and organs [10]. Among all the various tissues and organs, tendons comprise collagen fibrils with unique hierarchical structures (**Figure 1**) that are responsible for human motor function [11]. Therefore, the fabrication of artificial tendons is a good example of biomaterials developed using aligned collagen fibrils as a structural backbone. As stated in this review, research on artificial tendons made using collagen has rapidly increased in the last decade to meet the clinical needs of replacing autologous tendon transplants.

Artificial tendons must have uniaxially aligned collagen fibrils running parallel to the geometrical axis; this characteristic collagen structure is responsible for the excellent mechanical features of live tendons [12]. Collagen fibrils can be simply prepared by well-known *in vitro* fibrillogenesis. Collagen molecules are stable in acidic solutions at low temperatures and are capable of self-assembling nanofibrils that respond to body temperature and neutral pH [13, 14]. The fibrils exhibit amorphous networks. Previous attempts to produce aligned fibril-based biomaterials used electrospinning, freeze drying, strong magnetic fields, and mechanical methods, such as shearing and tension during wet extrusion. Of these, only mechanical methods demonstrated the potential for use in the industrial production of artificial tendons by showing the ability to maintain and hierarchize collagen fibril structures.

Although many reviews on the fabrication of aligned collagen fibrils have been published in recent years [15–17], they do not focus on mechanical methods and the fabrication mechanisms therein. Here, we introduce the various mechanical methods of producing biomaterials with aligned collagen fibrils and discuss their mechanism and limitations in detail. This review will also act as a significant introduction for researchers willing to apply collagen-based artificial tendons in clinical practice.

2. Requirements of collagen-based artificial tendons

Tendon tissues connect muscles to bones and influence the transmission of mechanical loads between them [12, 18]. Ligament tissues connect bone to bone and stabilize joints [12, 18]. These two types of tissues are similar in structure and comprise uniaxially aligned collagen fibrils [19]. The characteristic structure of tendons and ligaments is a multi-unit hierarchical structure comprising longitudinally aligned collagen molecules (approximately 1 nm in diameter), fibrils (approximately 100 nm in diameter), fibers (1–20 μm in diameter), and fascicles (20–200 μm in diameter) [11]. This hierarchical organization of collagen fibrils is crucial to the nonlinear and viscoelastic mechanical properties of collagen-based organs [20]. Tendons and ligaments are remarkable for their superior tensile strength and stiffness; the tensile strengths of the Achilles' tendon and anterior cruciate ligament (ACL) are 54 ± 20 MPa [21] and 24 ± 9 MPa [22], respectively, and their tensile moduli are 212 ± 109 MPa [21] and 113 ± 45 MPa [22], respectively.

Tendons and ligaments are tough tissues; however, ruptures of these tissues are common traumas among athletes [23]. The ACL is a part of a pair of cruciate ligaments (the other being the posterior cruciate ligament) in the human knee that connects the femur to the tibia to stabilize knee joint movements. ACL is the most frequently injured knee ligament [24]. Once the ACL ruptures, it can rarely connect end-to-end through conservative treatments. The poor healing capacity of ACL, particularly after rupture, is clinically common, although the underlying reasons for this remain unclear [25]. ACL reconstruction surgeries are required for such traumas; ACL injuries are among the most common among the athletic populations, with nearly 130,000 ACL reconstructions performed in 2006 in the USA alone [26]. Although there are no published survey results, ACL construction surgeries in Japan are estimated to exceed 17,000 per year.

In recent years, autogenous tendon tissues have been frequently used as substitutes for human tendon grafts (allografts) to reconstruct torn ligaments [27]. One notable advantage of this reconstruction surgery is the remodeling property of the autogenous tendon [28, 29], called ligamentization. Although the process of biological remodeling remains incompletely understood, clinicians agree that the strength of an autogenous tendon graft reduces soon after reconstruction and gradually increases with time, accompanied by structural changes in the collagen fibers [30]. Intrinsic fibroblasts in the tendon graft undergo ischemic necrosis followed by extrinsic cell infiltration with graft revascularization [31]. After remodeling implanted autogenous tendon tissues, patients can return to their daily activities as before. However, autogenous tendon grafting inevitably results in damage and consequent morbidity at the donor site, necessitating a second invasive procedure [32]. Although allogenous tendons are considered an alternative graft material, they have their disadvantages, including disease transmission risk and slow graft remodeling [33]. Currently, tendon xenografts cannot be used in a clinical setting; accordingly, synthetic tendons have been studied to avoid these disadvantages [16]. Various synthetic materials, such as polyethylene and polytetrafluoroethylene, have been used previously to create artificial tendons. However, they have not been clinically used as they fail after implantation because they undergo biodegradation without any remodeling [34]. Therefore, the fabrication of artificial tendons showing hierarchical structures of uniaxially aligned collagen fibrils seems to be the most promising approach as they are expected to undergo remodeling in the human body after implantation in a manner similar to that of autogenous tendon tissues [16, 19].

3. Overview of the fabrication methods used for aligned collagen fibrils

3.1 Electrospinning

Before focusing on the mechanical methods, we present an overview of the fabrication methods used for aligning collagen fibrils. Electrospinning has been widely considered an efficient method for fabricating polymer nanofibers, and several studies have described this fabrication technique [35, 36]. Briefly, the system comprises three elements—polymer solutions dissolved in volatile solvents, a high voltage supplier, and a metal target. The high voltage supplier provides electric potential differences in many kV between the polymer solutions and the target. The polymer solutions are then gradually extruded through a needle, and the electrically charged polymer solution is ejected from the tip of the needle which then reaches the target while being spun into thin threads (in the order of nm to μm in diameter). The volatile solvents evaporate during the interim, resulting in the collection of the polymer nanofiber mesh.

When the target is rotated during collagen electrospinning, each nanofiber tends to be aligned uniaxially [37]. Such materials can be helpful in *in vitro* experiments that evaluate the effects of scaffold alignments on the biological behaviors of cultured cells [37–39]. However, electrospinning appears to be an ineffective option as a fabrication method for artificial tendons due to the inevitable collagen denaturation. Fluoroalcohols are used as solvents to dissolve the collagen as this hydrophilic polymer shows little or no solubility in conventional volatile solvents for electrospinning, such as dichloromethane and chloroform. Zeugolis et al. demonstrated that collagen in electrospun nanofibers was denatured to gelatin almost completely using fluoroalcohols as solvents [40]. This event can be explained by the ability of fluoroalcohols to break hydrogen bonds among proteins. A pioneering study of collagen electrospinning [41] demonstrated a characteristic cross-striated pattern of collagen fibrils in electrospun nanofibers fabricated using hexafluoroisopropanol as a solvent; however, the debris of collagen fibrils is presumed to have remained according to the findings of Zeugolis et al. The nanofibers prepared using electrospinning collagen solutions cannot be defined as collagen nanofibers.

3.2 Freeze drying

Freeze drying (also called freeze-casting) is one of the most critical industrial processes used to preserve heat-sensitive biological materials, including food, pharmaceuticals, microorganisms, and plants, with minimal deterioration of their intrinsic chemical and physical properties during the drying processes [42]. The fundamental principle of freeze drying is sublimation, that is, the direct shift from a solid state to a gaseous state [43]. The freeze drying process can be explained through a characteristic phase diagram of solid (ice), liquid (water), and gas (vapor). When water-based slurry, suspension, or solution is frozen at atmospheric pressure, the contents in water are separated from ice crystals and concentrated. If we increase the temperature of the frozen material above 0°C while keeping the atmospheric pressure below 0.06 atm, the ice turns into a gas without going through a liquid phase in accordance with the phase diagram of water [43]. Generally, dried materials thus obtained have microporous structures, whereas the contents eliminated from the ice crystals had thin walls and pores, which was similar to that of ice crystals [44].

Based on the above freeze-drying principle, Schoof et al. fabricated collagen sponges using aligned structures of pores and thin walls using the unidirectional solidification technique [45, 46]. Briefly, a cylindrical container filled with a collagen suspension was sandwiched from the top and bottom using a pair of copper blocks and then cooled with liquid nitrogen. Plate-like ice grew in the collagen suspension along the depth of the cylindrical container, by which collagen molecules are eliminated from the unidirectional solidification of the growing ice crystals. Freeze drying the frozen suspension created unidirectional thin collagen walls and interconnected pores. The pores had a width of 20–40 μm and were alternately separated by much thinner walls; this structure can be considered as collagen fibers with wide gaps. Some researchers have thus used unidirectional solidification to fabricate fibers from suspensions of collagen molecules or fibrils [47–49]. Additionally, a modified technique has been developed to concentrate collagen axially and form a fiber-like construct [50]. As a result, those macromolecules are likely to be partially aligned because of the high aspect ratios. However, there is little evidence of the unidirectional alignment of collagen fibrils in the walls after freeze drying, whereas aligned thin walls or fiber-like structures were observed microscopically [45–49]. The authors believe that collagen in the micro structures is almost amorphous on a fibrillar scale, affecting cellular responses and morphologies.

3.3 Exposure to a strong magnetic field

Based on the fact that some proteins in solutions exhibit birefringence under strong magnetic fields, Torbet et al. demonstrated for the first time that collagen fibrils are magnetically aligned [51]. A neutral collagen solution (0.6 mg/mL) was heated from 4°C to 27.5°C to induce fibrillogenesis under a strong magnetic field (13T), resulting in the formation of aligned collagen fibrils. Collagen molecules have a negative diamagnetic anisotropy and they lie perpendicular to the magnetic field. Many researchers have applied this method to fabricate aligned collagen fibril hydrogels and used the gels for *in vitro* examinations to assess the effects of collagen fibril alignments on cell behaviors [52–56].

The notable advantage of this strong magnetic field is that it is noninvasive to living cells and organisms. However, the disadvantage is the lack of mass productivity of tough collagen fibers. The starting substance of the fabrication process is a neutral collagen solution, which is set in a narrow chamber (a few cm) with a strong magnetic field generator. This small-batch process is not suitable for the mass production of biomaterials. Further, the concentration of the collagen solution has to be low enough (≤10 mg/mL) to allow the rotation of the molecules due to magnetic force, preventing the production of high-density collagen fibrils. Recently, new methods have been developed wherein magnetic substances (beads or rods) are added to collagen solutions to mechanically pull or assist in the alignment of collagen fibril under magnetic fields [57–60]. A challenge associated with these manufacturing methods is that the magnetic substances are retained in the collagen gel.

3.4 Electrochemical method

Electrochemical fabrication for assembling aligned collagen bundles was first reported in 2008 [61]. This method is substantially different from the previous method using strong magnetic fields in that the physical force does not directly affect the collagen molecules. When the parallel set anode and cathode electrodes are soaked in a shallow pool of collagen solution, a pH gradient perpendicular to the electrodes is generated by the migration of electrolytes. Collagen molecules with a low pH are positively charged, whereas those with high pH are negatively charged. Therefore, all the collagen molecules migrate toward the isoelectric point (pH 8.2), congregate, and form fibrils under neutral conditions. The electrochemically aligned collagen (ELAC) threads with diameters of 50–400 μm and lengths of 3–7 cm were prepared depending on the electrodes used [61]. Although electron microscopies have not yet visualized uniaxial alignments of collagen fibrils, it is reasonable that collagen fibrils tend to align uniaxially by the electrochemical compaction to a bundle.

Continuous molding of ELAC threads was successfully performed using a rotating electrode electrochemical alignment device [62]. The main parts of the device include a power supply for providing voltage for the electrochemical cell, a syringe pump, a rotating electrodes wheel, and a collection spool. A collagen solution is extruded onto the caved edge of the rotating electrodes wheel placed vertically. The electrodes are placed parallel on the wheel's edge, allowing continuous ELAC formation synchronized with the rotation speed. Furthermore, ELAC threads were twisted to form yarn, and the yarn was pin-weaved toward a highly porous scaffold as an artificial tendon. The ELAC scaffolds showed ultimate stress and tensile modulus comparable to the natural tendon [62]. Furthermore, the biological effects of collagen fibril alignments in ELAC threads have been assessed *in vitro* [62–66] and *in vivo* [67].

The electrochemical method is the first to continuously produce aligned collagen fibril threads. ELAC threads (diameters 50–400 μm) in the yarns seem to correspond to collagen fibers (diameters ~20 μm [11]) in living tendons, although the diameters of the former are much larger. Further studies are required for ELAC thread-based biomaterials to provide the tendon-like hierarchical structure of collagen fibrils.

3.5 Mechanical methods

The main purpose of this paper is to describe the mechanism and challenges associated with manufacturing tendon-like bundles of uniaxially aligned collagen fibrils through mechanical methods. Briefly, mechanical methods involve the use of mechanical force (shearing or tension) to align collagen fibrils. Mechanical forces can be generated before, during, or after the fibrillogenesis of collagen molecules.

4. Solution extrusion methods

Among the various aligned collagen fibril fabrication methods, mechanical methods have been extensively studied because of their simplicity and effectiveness as well as mass production suitability. These mechanical methods can be generally categorized into the following based on their fabrication mechanisms: solution extrusion methods (wet spinning and others), shear flow deposition, flow-induced crystallization, and gel-extrusion method. Herein, fabrication mechanism, effectiveness, and challenges of solution extrusion methods are discussed.

4.1 Wet spinning

Wet spinning is a typical example of a solution extrusion method that was first developed to produce collagen threads for artificial tendons [68]. A collagen solution is extruded from a narrow channel directly into a coagulation bath to form a cord-like gel through collagen fibril formation [69]. **Figure 2** shows a schematic illustration of a typical experimental setting for wet spinning. Neutral buffers such as phosphate buffer saline (PBS) containing polyethylene glycol (PEG) have been frequently used as coagulation baths for wet spinning as PBS provides suitable conditions for collagen fibrillogenesis [14] and PEG dehydrates the collagen molecules to promote fibrillogenesis. In Kato's method [68], the acidic collagen solution is filled in a reservoir, such as a syringe, and is extruded through a narrow tube (≤1 mm diameter) at a constant speed using a pump. The tip of the tube is submerged in a coagulation bath, and the collagen solution stream is immediately gelled due to fibrillogenesis. As a result, the cord-like collagen gel is continuously molded. Finally, drying the cord-like gel results

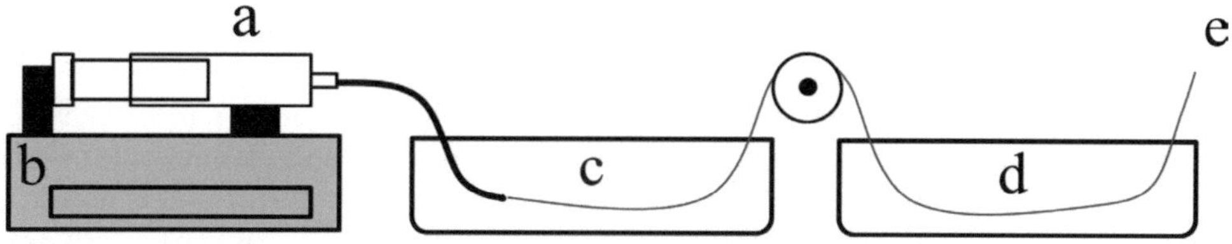

Figure 2.
Schematic illustration of the typical experimental setting for wet spinning. An acidic collagen solution in a syringe (a) is loaded in a syringe pump (b) and infused via a narrow tubing into a coagulation bath (neutral buffer containing PEG is frequently used) heated at 37°C (c). As a result, the cord-like collagen gel is continuously molded and sequentially introduced into an ethanol bath (d) to promote dehydration. The cord-like gel is then wound up and air-dried to produce a collagen thread (e).

in a tough thread with a diameter of 20–300 μm [70]. Cavallaro et al. succeeded in continuously processing dried collagen threads through a sequence of conventional wet spinning and subsequent drying using a ventilation-type cabinet [71]. Acetone was also used as a coagulation bath, allowing the fabrication of narrow collagen threads with an approximate diameter of 15 μm [72].

After Kato's pioneer study, many researchers have applied wet spinning to fabricate collagen threads for different biomaterials [69, 73]. However, the nanostructures of the collagen threads fabricated by wet spinning are far from those of tendon unit structures. Pins *et al.* revealed that collagen fibrils in wet spun threads were amorphous, prompting alignment by stretching the wet spun threads [74]. Despite many studies on wet spinning, the molecular events in the thread-making process have not yet been clarified, but it is likely that oriented collagen molecules under shearing in a narrow channel immediately changed to amorphous after extrusion into a coagulation bath (discussed in Section 4.5).

Assuming that the rapid relaxation of the oriented collagen molecules occurs, some treatments for delaying relaxation effectively promote fibril alignments in wet spinning. The addition of viscous materials or increase in collagen concentration to delay collagen molecule relaxation prior to fibrillogenesis has been investigated. Nerger et al. investigated 3-D bioprinting of collagen ink containing LAPONITE® (a type of layered silicate), Pluronic® F-127 (a type of polyethylene glycol), or Matrigel® (extracellular matrices of sarcoma) as rheology-adjusting agents [75]. The cord-like collagen gel extruded from a conical nozzle comprised of incompletely but preferably aligned collagen fibrils. Lai et al. prepared 30 mg/mL of rat tail collagen solution by dialysis against PEG and used it for fabricating tubular collagen gels with a custom-made syringe [76]. The fibrils on the surface of the collagen gels were aligned almost uniaxially, whereas the alignments of interior fibrils were not observed.

4.2 Modified wet spinning

In 2010, Caves et al. attempted to increase the fibril alignment of wet spun fibers by dropping the extruded cord-like collagen gels vertically with a coagulation buffer [77]. The extrusion of the collagen solution into a coagulation bath was performed in the same manner as wet spinning, resulting in the continuous formation of a cord-like gel. The bath was a long column through which the coagulation buffer was circulated to generate a vertical flow for carrying the collagen gel downwards along the column while simultaneously stretching it. The fibril alignment in the dried collagen thread was higher than that obtained using conventional wet spinning [73]; however, mechanical stretching (strain ratio of 10–20%) was required to achieve uniaxial alignments.

Recently, an extrusion method has been developed that incorporates the sequential stretching process of extruded gels to overcome the lack of fibril alignments [78]. This experimental setting is illustrated in **Figure 3A**. The collagen solution was continuously introduced into a flat flow channel (1-mm thick and 35-mm wide) with a pair of buffers containing PEG to ensure the three-layer of buffer-collagen-buffer. During co-extrusion, the collagen solution could be coagulated to some extent by dehydration with PEG. A sheet-shaped stream of partially coagulated collagen solution was extruded from the outlet into a coagulation buffer, resulting in the continuous production of a collagen gel sheet. Subsequently, the gel sheet was stretched along the machine direction with a rotating mandrel, thus enhancing the alignment of the collagen fibrils. Finally, wet collagen sheets as thin as 1.9 μm were obtained

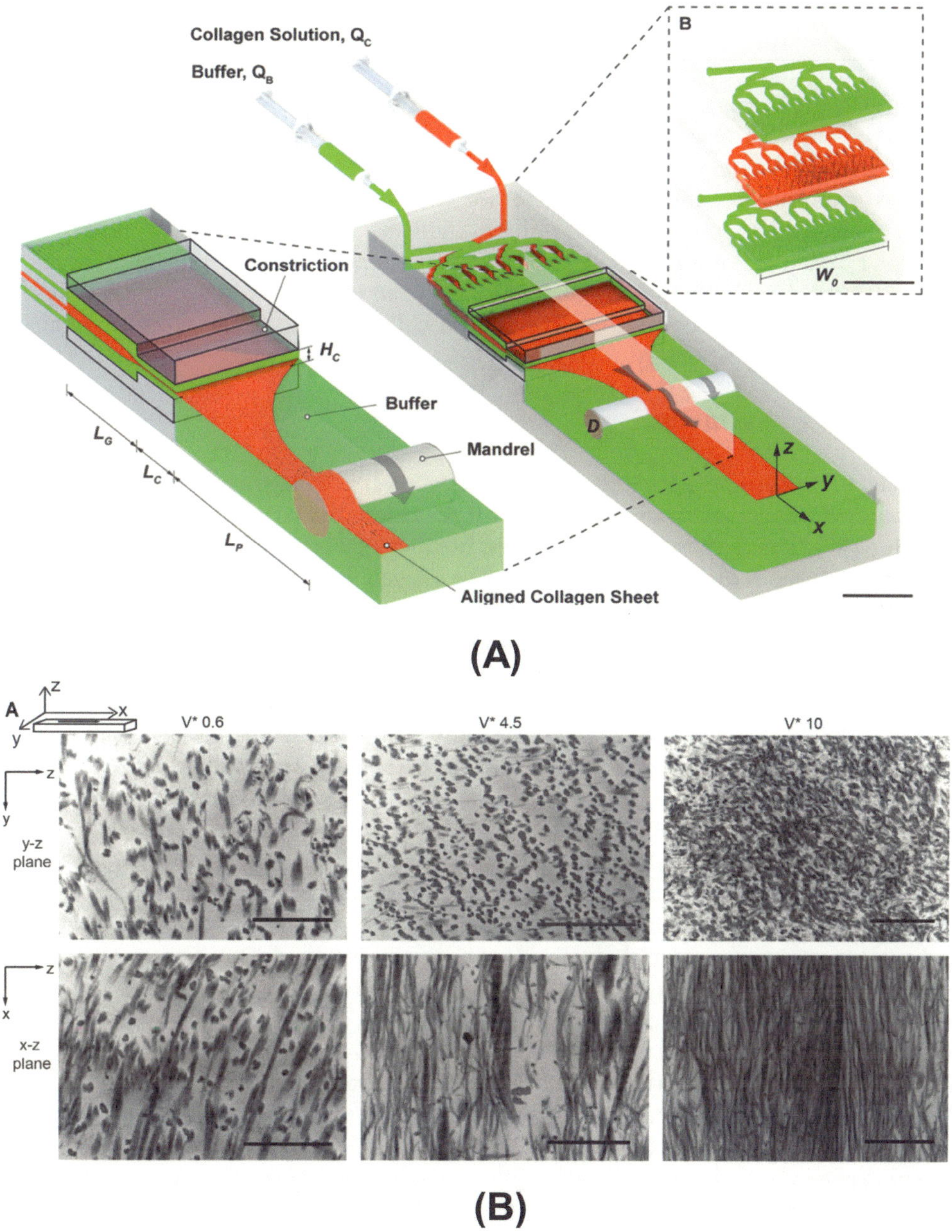

(A)

(B)

Figure 3.
Schematic illustration of the extrusion method incorporating sequential stretching of extruded sheet-shaped gels (A) and nanostructure of collagen gels observed on transmission electron microscopy (TEM) (B). (A) Collagen (red) and buffer solutions (green) are delivered to a three-layered microfluidic device. An emerging collagen sheet then undergoes fibrillogenesis and is strained by passing over a rotating mandrel. (B) TEM images of collagen sheets were produced at V of 0.6, 4.5, and 10 in (y − z) and (x − z) planes (depicted in (A)). V* = (Vp − VT)/VT, where Vp is the velocity of the rotating mandrel and VT is the total bulk velocity of the solutions passing through the flow constriction. Reproduced from Ref. [78] with permission from ACS Publication.*

which exhibited good mechanical qualities (tensile strength, 0.5–2.7 MPa and elastic moduli, 3–36 MPa). The alignment of collagen fibrils along the machine direction was enhanced depending on the rotating speed of the mandrel (**Figure 3B**).

Malladi's study indicates that the stretching process of extruded collagen gels can be incorporated into the conventional extrusion processes, including wet spinning. The stretching of gels was effective for enhancing the alignments of collagen fibrils, whereas fibrils extruded in the gels were almost amorphous. A parameter $V^* = (Vp - VT)/VT$ was used, where Vp is the velocity of the rotating mandrel and VT is the total bulk velocity of the solutions passing through the flow constriction. The elastic moduli increased as V^* increased from 0.1 to 10; this was explained by the fibril density and degree of fibril alignment increase. As per the authors' experience, collagen fibrillar gels are less stretchable. The excellent stretchability in this case ($V^* \leq 10$) could be due to the use of acid-solubilized rat tail tendon collagen [77] with intact intermolecular crosslinking. The type of collagen used in the experiment also affects the molding propriety.

4.3 Other extrusion methods

Lai et al. reported a fabrication method for cord-like collagen gels with longitudinally aligned fibrils effectively using shear force compared with a conventional wet spinning [79]. This method would result in fibrillogenesis [13, 14] before the relaxation of the shear force-induced orientation of the collagen molecules. An acidic collagen solution of rat tail tendon collagen (30 mg/mL) was continuously extruded from a syringe with a 22-gage needle onto a glass slide and submerged in a coagulation bath of 10× PBS. In this process, the syringe and glass slides were moved in opposite directions, thus generating shear forces on the extruded collagen solution, which immediately initiated fibrillogenesis while maintaining alignments of collagen molecules due to the solution's high viscosity, resulting in a cord-like collagen gel with aligned fibrils. When the human dermal microvascular endothelial cells were cultured on the gels, the cells exhibited elongated morphologies along the alignment direction of fibrils.

A method for producing edible collagen casings, that is, artificial intestine for sausage, [80] has been applied for manufacturing tubular gels comprising aligned collagen fibrils through a counter-rotating extrusion method [81, 82]. The experimental setting and appearance of the material obtained are shown in **Figure 4** [81]. This method does not include collagen fibrillogenesis but uses a fibril-rich collagen dough made from living tissues as a starting substrate. Briefly, the homogenized collagen dough (5% [w/v]) was fed to a metering pump and then into a counter-rotating extruder using a piston stuffer. This unique extruder comprises two coaxial cylinders rotating in the opposite direction. The collagen dough is continuously introduced into the gap (0.5 mm) between the larger and smaller cylinders along the axes of the cylinders so that the rotation in the opposite direction generates a shear force on the collagen dough in the gap. Consequently, tube-shaped collagen gels are extruded in which the collagen fibrils are preferably aligned in the circumferential direction. Thus, the tubes must be cut in the circumferential direction to fabricate an artificial tendon with longitudinally aligned fibrils.

The solution extrusion methods are summarized as follows: collagen molecules can be oriented using shear force in a narrow channel, resulting in the production of cord-like collagen gels with nearly amorphous fibrils. This is probably due to the immediate relaxation of the molecules after extrusion from the tips of the channels. Additional mechanical stretching is required to improve the alignment. Thus, suppression of molecular relaxation appears to be effective for fabricating collagen gels with longitudinally aligned fibrils. The use of collagen fibril dough as starting substances or the sequential stretching of gels is also effective.

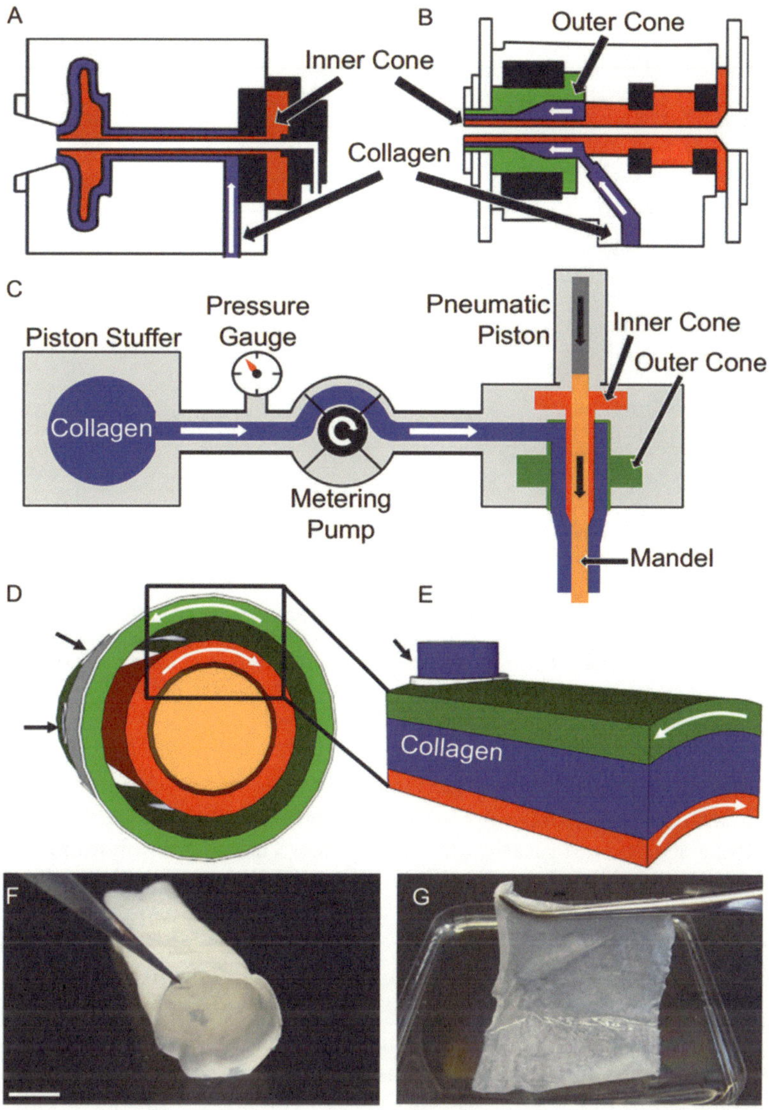

Figure 4.
Overview of counter-rotating extrusion method. (A–E) Schematic illustrations of the method. (F and G) Appearances of tube-shaped collagen gels obtained using this method. Reproduced from Ref. [81] with permission from Elsevier.

4.4 Limitations of solution extrusion methods

As described in Section 4.1, wet spinning has a limited capability of producing threads with well-aligned collagen fibrils, especially in the interior of threads. Although the mechanisms of solution extrusion have not been described in detail compared with those of shear flow deposition, it is obvious that rheological features of collagen solutions play a predominant role in the alignment of collagen fibrils. Here, rheological data of collagen solutions are introduced in the next paragraph to discuss the presumed mechanisms of solution extrusion.

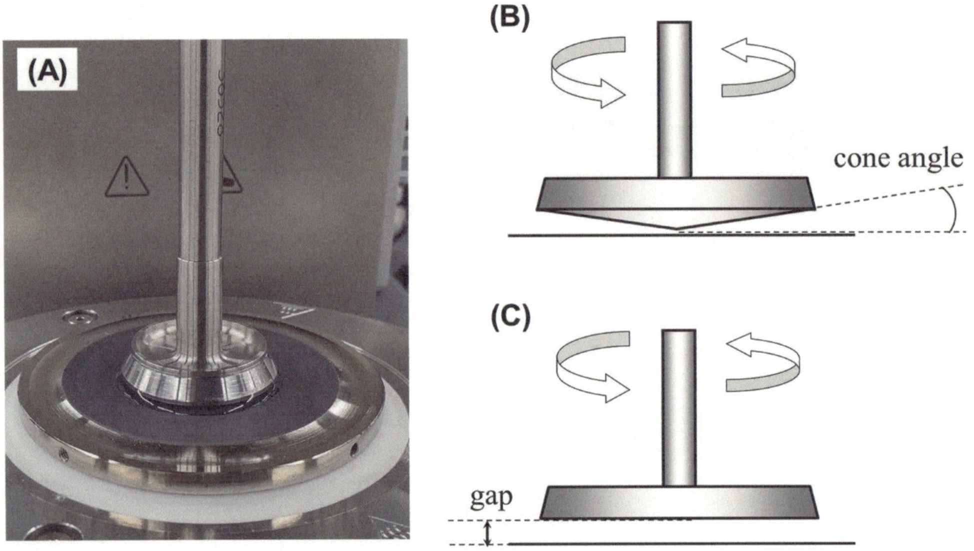

Figure 5.
Sensors of the rotational rheometer. (A) Appearance of a parallel plate sensor. (B) and (C) are schematic illustrations of cone plate and parallel plate sensor, respectively. A sample solution is placed on the Peltier-controlled bottom plate and the movable upper sensor is positioned to achieve a pre-set gap. The sensor is rotated unidirectionally to obtain rotational measurements. Oscillational measurements are obtained by sinusoidal oscillation with extremely small shear deformation (usually ≤1%).

For the rheological measurements, a rotational rheometer was used (MCR 502; Anton Paar, Ostfildern, Germany). This apparatus is effective for simultaneously evaluating the viscosity and gelation features of low viscous biopolymer solutions [83]. A collagen solution was filled in a gap between a Peltier-controlled bottom plate and a movable upper sensor (cone plate sensor, diameter, 35 mm; cone angle, 1°; parallel plate sensor, diameter, 50 mm) (**Figure 5**). This apparatus can conduct rotational as well as oscillational measurements. Rotational measurements measure the flow and viscosity curves of the specimen, providing information about reductions in increased shear stress (shear thinning) and thixotropic properties under shearing. Conversely, oscillational measurements are helpful in tracking the changing rheological properties of a collagen solution (in this case, recovery of rheological properties just after shearing). Two types of collagen were used, acid-solubilized collagen from the porcine tendon (designated ASC) (Cellmatrix® type I-A; 0.3% solution, Nitta Gelatin, Osaka, Japan) and pepsin-digested collagen from the porcine dermis (designated PC) (Collagen BM; 0.53% solution, Nitta Gelatin, Osaka, Japan). ASC remains intermolecular crosslinking, and the physicochemical qualities can be considered as similar to those of a conventional rat tail tendon collagen. PC is a representative of pepsin-digested collagens which are generally used for commercial biomedical devices.

Rotational measurements simulated the behaviors of collagen molecules during wet spinning processes. **Figure 6** presents the viscosity curves of collagen solutions obtained by reciprocal rotational measurements at shear rates 0.1–100 s^{-1}. Both the collagen solutions showed a shear rate-dependent decrease in viscosities (non-Newtonian behavior) during the shear rate-rising process, suggesting molecular alignments along the flow direction. The viscosity curves obtained from the falling of shear rates overlapped almost entirely in both the collagens, suggesting that the alignments of collagen molecules under shearing are not hysteresis. A sequential

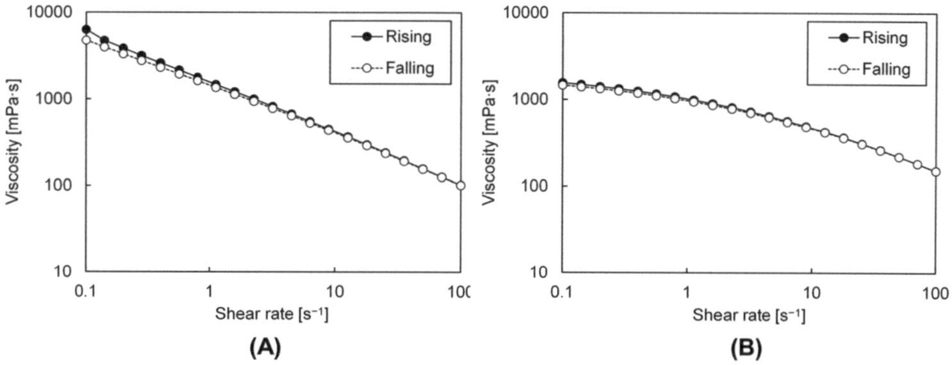

Figure 6.
Viscosity curves of collagen solutions were obtained by reciprocal rotational measurements at shear rates of 0.1–100 s^{-1}. (A) Acid-solubilized collagen from porcine tendon (0.3%) and (B) pepsin-digested collagen from porcine dermis (0.53%). Both the solutions showed a shear rate-dependent decrease in viscosities (non-Newtonian behavior) during the shear rate-rising process. The viscosity curves obtained from the falling of shear rates overlapped almost entirely in both the collagens.

test of oscillation-rotation-oscillation was used (**Figure 7**) to simulate conditions of collagen molecules in wet spinning. The first step is the oscillational measurement at constant shear deformation (1%) and frequency (1 Hz) to test the viscoelastic qualities of the collagen solution as a starting substance wherein collagen molecules are dispersed amorphously. The rapid rotation (shear rate, 100 s^{-1}) as the second step

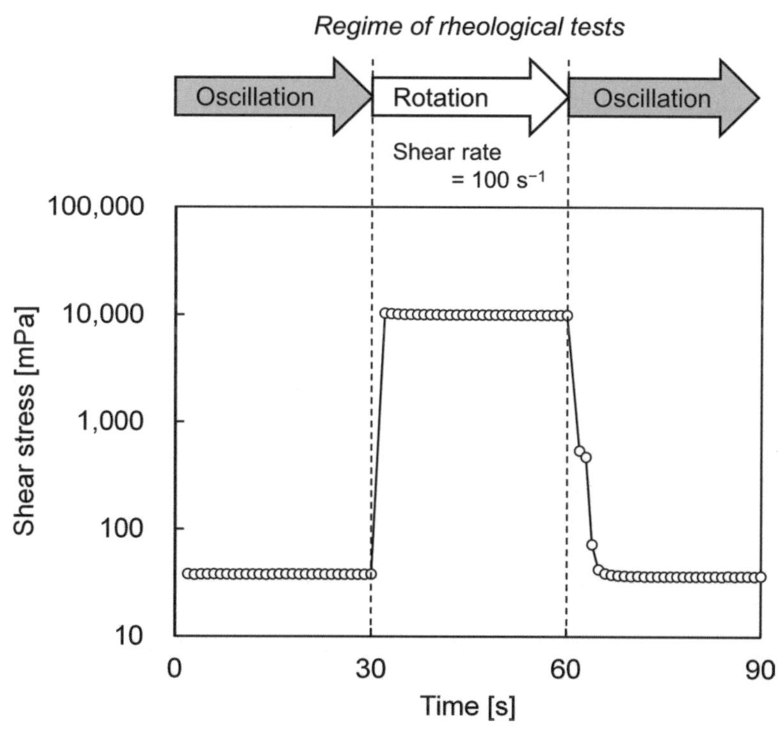

Figure 7.
Scheme and results of sequential testing of oscillation–rotation–oscillation for evaluating the relaxation of collagen molecules.

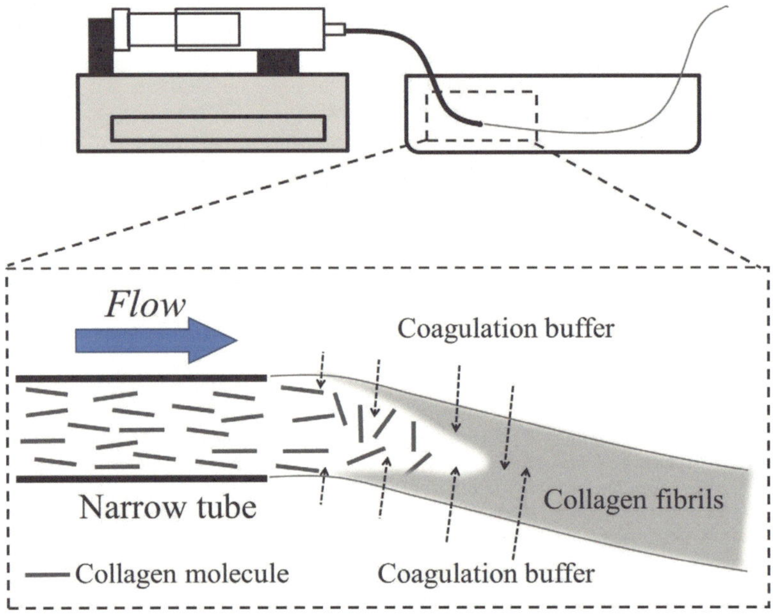

Figure 8.
Schematic illustration of a conceivable scenario in the thread-making process of wet spinning. An acidic collagen solution is extruded through a narrow tube, in which collagen molecules should be oriented along the flow direction. The stream of the viscous collagen solution extruded from the tip of the tube should immediately coagulate to form fibrils from the surface layer. If the coagulant penetrates the stream of the collagen solution before the molecular orientation is relaxed, the collagen fibrils are aligned. However, the alignments of collagen molecules would be immediately relaxed and become amorphous.

simulates strong shearing on the collagen solution introduced into a narrow tube. Oscillational measurement as the last step monitors the recovery of shear stress after the collagen solution is released from the strong shearing, which can simulate the recovery of amorphous dispersion of collagen molecules just after extrusion into a coagulation bath. **Figure 7** indicates the results of the sequential test for ASC. The shear stress sharply decreased by more than one order of magnitude (from 9940 mPa to 540 mPa) only in 2 s after the rotation was terminated and subsequently became identical to that obtained at the first step (before rotational shearing). The small delay in the recovery of shear stress could be due to the inertial force of the flowing collagen solution.

Considering this rapid recovery of shear stress and no hysteresis of viscosity curves, the following scenario is conceivable in the thread-making process of wet spinning (**Figure 8**). An acidic collagen solution is extruded through a narrow tube wherein the collagen molecules should be oriented preferably along the flow direction, as proposed from the non-Newtonian behavior of an acidic collagen solution (**Figure 6**). The stream of the viscous collagen solution extruded from the tip of the tube should immediately coagulate to form fibrils on the surface layer. If the coagulant penetrates the stream of the collagen solution before the molecular orientation is relaxed, the collagen fibrils are aligned. However, the alignment of collagen molecules with an approximate molecular weight of 300,000 will be immediately relaxed and become amorphous, as suggested by the stress-relaxation curves of an acidic collagen solution (**Figure 7**). The above scenario somewhat explains the mechanism of collagen fibril alignments in the solution extrusion methods.

5. Other mechanical methods

The previous paragraph described wet spinning and other solution extrusion methods derived from wet spinning. In the last decade, unique mechanical methods were newly developed to fabricate biomaterials with aligned collagen fibrils. Herein, the fabrication mechanism, effectiveness, and challenges of other mechanical methods (shear flow deposition, flow-induced crystallization, and gel-extrusion method) are discussed.

5.1 Shear flow deposition

This section focuses on the methods of applying shear force during collagen fibrillogenesis, called shear flow deposition. When some part of a collagen fibril is anchored onto a substrate under a strong shear flow, the fibrils are aligned in the direction of flow. This investigation is conducted using a thin collagen solution with low viscosity and a thin flow channel to induce a uniform and fast flow.

In 2009, Saeidi et al. reported the effects of shear rates on fibril alignments in the shear flow deposition using a microfluidic shear flow chamber [84], which can generate a wide range of shear rates. They examined the detailed dynamics of neutralized pepsin-extracted type I collagen assembly on a glass surface under the influence of shear flow between two plates. Differential interference contrast imaging with focal plane stabilization was used to resolve and track the growth of collagen aggregates on borosilicate glass under various shear rates (500, 80, 20, and 9 s^{-1}). The nucleation of fibrils on the glass was observed to occur rapidly (~2 min) followed by the continued growth of the fibrils. The best alignment of fibrils was observed at intermediate shear rates of 20 and 80 s^{-1}, whereas the growth rates were affected by the shear rate in a complex manner. However, the investigation showed that directional fibril growth was not stable and the fibrils would often turn downstream, forming "hooks" at high shear rates.

In Saeidi's next study [85], a spin-coating technique was combined with a flow of collagen solution to produce highly aligned arrays of collagen fibrils. A chilled neutral collagen solution was introduced into the center of the spin coater, which was heated to initiate collagen fibrillogenesis. Orthogonal collagen lamellae were successfully fabricated on the coater depending on shear rates (181–2480 s^{-1}), which were adjusted by flow rates (0.1–1 mL/min) and rotation speeds (750–3000 rpm). It was possible to produce small sections (1 cm^2) of collagen fibrils with enough alignment to guide fibroblasts. However, thin-film instabilities on the coater are likely to be a significant barrier to manufacturing organized collagen fibrils over larger areas.

The effects of planar substrates with collagen-binding features on shear flow deposition were evaluated by Lanfer et al. [86]. They used a microfluidic channel system with coverslip substrates coated with poly(octadecene-alt-maleic acid) (POMA), which could bind collagen fibrils. The aligned collagen fibrils were successfully deposited on the substrates, where the degree of collagen fibril alignment increased with increasing flow rates of the solution. The matrix density increased at higher collagen solution concentrations and on hydrophobic polymer pre-coatings.

The shear flow deposition can deposit well-aligned fibrils on substrates, thus providing some insights into the fabrication conditions for achieving tendon-like collagen fibrillar gels. However, there is a limitation to fabricating thick and long products of aligned collagen fibrils. Collagen fibrils can be anchored directly to substrates at the beginning of the fabrication, promoting fibril alignments along the shear flow direction. However, in the following steps, collagen fibrils cannot be deposited due to the lack of binding features between collagen fibrils. Shear flow deposition methods are likely to be helpful in fabricating cell culture substrates rather than therapeutic biomaterials, such as artificial tendons, to investigate the effects of collagen anisotropy on the biological behaviors of living cells [87, 88].

5.2 Flow-induced crystallization

Before describing flow-induced crystallization, the capacity of collagen molecules to form liquid crystalline should be described. At a molecular level, acid-soluble collagen molecules spontaneously assemble into precholesteric-banded patterns and cholesteric phases at concentrations above 50 mg/mL [89]. Stabilization of the liquid crystalline collagen, induced by pH modification and resultant fibrillogenesis, indicates characteristic morphologies of collagen fibril arrays in bone tissues. Furthermore, a dense gel (18 wt%) prepared by self-reassembly of collagen molecules *in vitro* shows characteristic bundles of cross-striated fibrils observed in the tendon. The qualities of collagen molecules imply that the formation of liquid crystalline at high concentrations is a key factor for manufacturing bundles of uniaxially aligned collagen fibrils.

In 2016, Paten et al. developed a novel fabrication method called flow-induced crystallization through which dense collagen molecules were microfluidically drawn to form a fiber of uniaxially aligned fibrils [90]. **Figure 9A** presents the schematic illustration of the fiber-making process. Briefly, a droplet of neutralized collagen solution was set under a flow of dry nitrogen gas, facilitating evaporation of water from the droplet surface and the formation of an enriched monomeric surface. A glass microneedle was used to pierce the droplet surface, and the dense collagen solution adhered to the tip of the needle. When the needle was drawn back to attain a low strain rate $< 1\ s^{-1}$), the surface collagen solution was pulled up to form a thread. In this processing, flow-induced crystallization and mechanical tension-induced fibril alignment could occur. Finally, a narrow fiber as a highly aligned collagen fibrillar array was created (**Figure 9B**).

Although the flow-induced crystallization method is still a form of microfluidic examination, each event in the processing provides us with ideas for creating uniaxially aligned collagen fibrils. When a dense collagen solution with the ability to form liquid crystalline is exposed to strong shearing or tension, the collagen molecules could be ready for uniaxial fibrillogenesis. Therefore, we have to consider the possibility of the continuous heating of the dense collagen solution under strong shearing or tension resulting in uniaxial fibrillogenesis. It is expected that a continuous fabrication of a thread of uniaxially aligned collagen fibrils is developed and scaled up based on the processing of Paten et al.

5.3 Gel-extrusion method

The last mechanical method for aligned collagen fibrils is the gel extrusion recently developed by the authors' group. This method can continuously fabricate cord-like collagen fibrillar gels by incorporating the advantages of the solution extrusion method and shear flow deposition. Those are continuous extrusion of collagen solution under shearing and simultaneous stretching of fibrils by shear force.

First, we evaluated the phenomenon caused by applying shear stress to collagen during fibrillogenesis using a rotational rheometer as a measuring device and a sample fabrication device [91]. A neutral collagen solution was filled in a gap between a Peltier-controlled bottom plate and a movable upper sensor (parallel plate sensor: diameter 60 mm). Fibrillogenesis under shearing occurred by increasing the

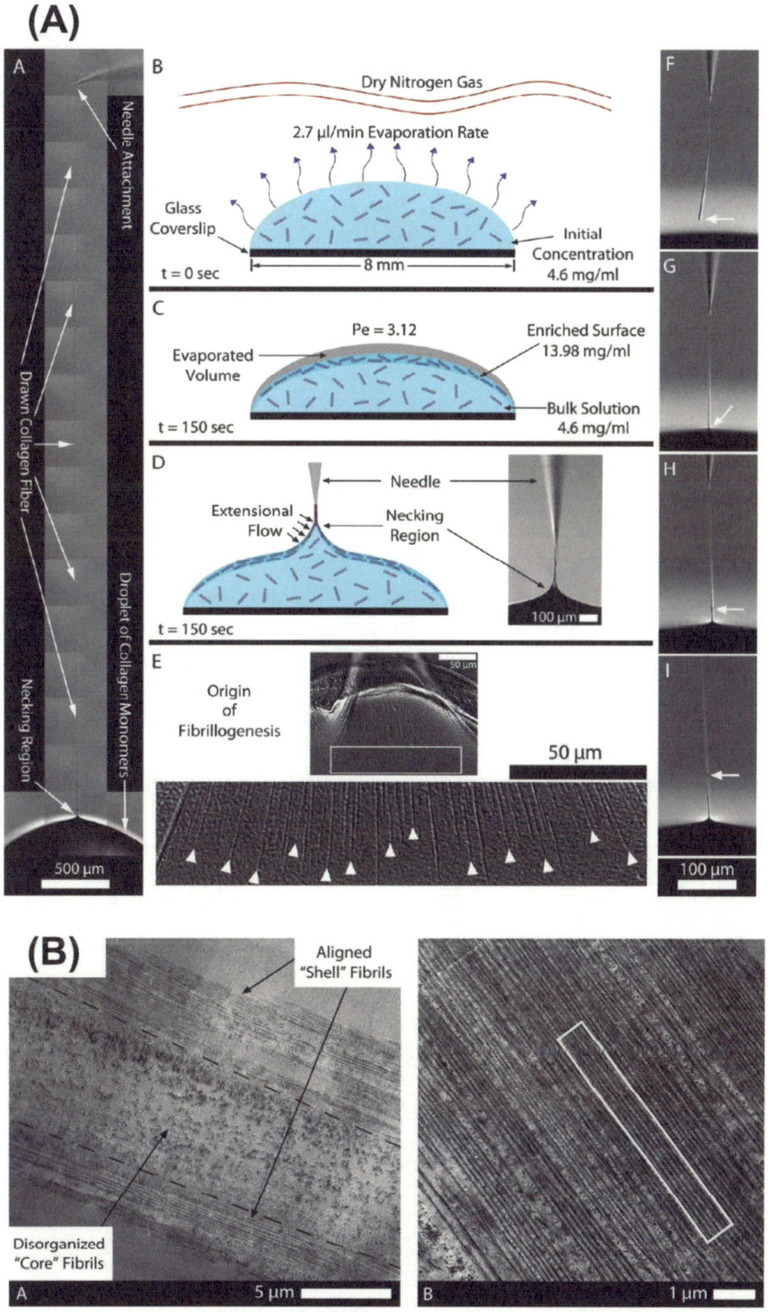

Figure 9.
Overview of flow-induced crystallization technique. (A) Schematic illustration and appearances of the fiber-making process. (B) Transmission electron microscopy images of the collagen fiber. Reproduced from Ref. [90] with permission from Elsevier.

temperature of the bottom plate (from 23 to 37°C) during rotation of the upper sensor. Wide ranges of collagen concentrations (0.1–2 wt %) and shear rates (0.1–500 s^{-1}) were preliminarily examined, but the gels were destroyed completely between the plate and sensor. The most crucial factor for successfully preparing gels under those conditions was the rate of fibrillogenesis gelation. Increased concentrations of neutral phosphate buffer could accelerate the gelation rate, and fibril alignment occurred within 20 s during the early stage of rapid gelation. Fabrication of gels was completed with slippage between gels and the movable upper plate, and well-aligned fibrils along the rotation direction were observed in the marginal regions of disk-shaped gels. Gel thickness could be increased from 1 mm to 3 mm with the homogeneous alignment of fibrils in the entire sample. The alignment of fibrils enhanced mechanical qualities against tensile loads placed parallel to the alignment axis. The elongation of cultured fibroblasts along the alignment was observed on the gels.

Next, a continuous formation method of cord-like collagen gels comprising fibrils preferentially aligned along the geometrical axes (CCGs) was developed by transferring the events on a rotational rheometer to those in a stainless tube [92]. The experimental setting was simple (**Figure 10A**). Collagen (2.5%) dissolved in a sodium phosphate buffer containing 280 mM sodium chloride was introduced into a stainless cylinder (length 52 mm, diameter 2.0 mm) heated to 38°C at a linear velocity of 2.5 mm s^{-1}. This process caused collagen fibril alignments under acute fibril formation in the cylinder, causing the continuous formation of CCGs (**Figure 10B**). Fibril formation rate, shear rate, and shear duration were substantial factors for successful CCG formation. Advantages of this method over conventional wet spinning include the capacity of this method to form aligned fibrils in the entire gels and to control the diameter of cord-like gels over 1 mm (**Figure 10C-10F**). The air-drying of CCGs, which were cross-linked with 1-ethyl-3-(3-dimethylaminopropyl)-carbodiimide and N-hydroxy-succinimide, produced dry collagen fibers with cross-sectional areas of 0.0123–0.135 mm^2 (**Figure 10G**). Upon the rewetting of the fibers, they failed at a stress of 54.5 ± 7.8 MPa, which is higher than the mean failure stress of ACL tissue (13.3–37.8 MPa). These findings show that the CCG formation method enables the fabrication of collagen fibers, which are potential components of collagen-based artificial tendons.

A limitation of the gel-extrusion method is the incomplete alignment of collagen fibrils along the geometrical axes, especially in the core region of the gel. The mechanism of fibril alignment could explain this heterogeneity, the process of alignment

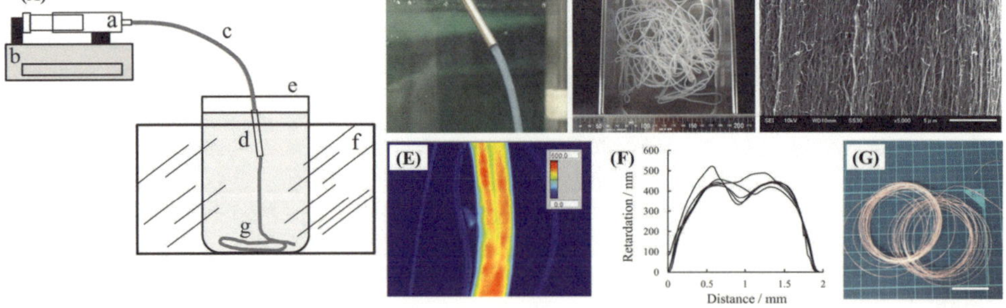

Figure 10.
Overview of the gel-extrusion method. (A) Schematic of the experimental setting. Collagen solution in a syringe (a) was loaded in a syringe pump (b) and infused via silicone tubing (c) into a stainless cylinder (d), which was immersed in a neutral buffer in a glass beaker (e) heated at 38°C in a water bath (f). A cord-like collagen gel was continuously extruded from the cylinder and accumulated on the bottom of the glass beaker (g). (B and C) A 2.0 mm diameter stainless steel cylinder during the processing and the stacked gels within. Longitudinal cross-sectional scanning electron microscopy images of the gel. Bar in figure indicates 5 μm. (E) Two-dimensional birefringence images of the gel. (F) Retardation of the gel across the perpendicular direction. (G) Appearance of dry fibers obtained from the cord-like gel. Bar in the figure indicates 20 mm.

of collagen fibrils involved their formation and then their immediate stretching by shear stress. The entanglement points act as anchors for stretching fibrils. The lengths of fibrils between entanglements were unequal, resulting in more and less stretched fibrils at a certain shear deformation. The stainless tube was heated in a water bath, causing a slower temperature elevation rate in the core region.

6. Conclusions

In conclusion, the mechanical methods for creating aligned collagen-based biomaterials are summarized. Previous attempts to fabricate uniaxially aligned fibrils have used electrospinning, freeze drying, strong magnetic field, electrochemical methods, along with mechanical methods, including shearing and tension during wet extrusion. Among the various fabrication methods, mechanical methods have been extensively studied because of their simplicity and effectiveness along with suitability for mass production. Mechanical methods can be generally divided into the following four methods depending on their fabrication mechanisms: solution extrusion methods (wet spinning and others), shear flow deposition, flow-induced crystallization, and gel-extrusion method. Solution extrusion methods can continuously mold cord-like collagen gels, from which collagen threads are prepared by air-drying. However, collagen fibrils in wet spun threads were amorphous, thus additional stretching of the threads is required to promote fibril alignments. The lack of fibril alignments is probably due to the immediate relaxation of the oriented molecules after the extrusion of collagen solutions. Additional mechanical stretching of gels or threads and delay of molecular relaxation in collagen solutions are effective to promote collagen fibril alignments. The use of collagen fibril dough as starting substance is also effective.

Shear flow deposition can deposit well-aligned fibrils on substrates. However, there is a limitation in fabricating thick and long products of aligned collagen fibrils. Collagen fibrils can be anchored directly to substrates at the beginning of the fabrication, promoting fibril alignments along the shear flow direction. But in the following steps, collagen fibrils cannot be deposited due to the lack of binding features between collagen fibrils.

Flow-induced crystallization is still a kind of microfluidic examination, combined with liquid crystallization of dense collagen solutions. This method can produce ultrathin threads of uniaxially aligned collagen fibrils. However, the production is not continuous because the starting substance is a partially dried surface of a droplet of collagen solution. It is expected that a continuous fabrication of collagen threads is developed and scaled up based on the processing of flow-induced crystallization.

The gel-extrusion method is a continuous formation method of cord-like collagen gels composed of fibrils preferably aligned along the geometrical axes in the entire gels. The feature of this method is the use of neutralized collagen sol, where the temperature-responsive fibrillogenesis is accelerated. The collagen sol is introduced into a heated channel where it can form fibrillar gels. The fibrils are aligned by shear force and stretching. A limitation of the gel-extrusion method is the incomplete alignment of collagen fibrils along the geometrical axes, especially in the core region of the gel.

Mechanical methods have recently made rapid progress. However, each of the methods cannot create artificial tendons with hierarchical structures of uniaxially aligned collagen fibrils with a capacity to undergo remodeling in the living body after implantation similar to autogenous tendon tissues. It is still challenging for biomaterial engineering to satisfy excellent mechanical and biological features. There are two promising approaches for creating an ideal collagen-based artificial tendon, bottom-up and top-down approaches. The bottom-up approach is the creation of collagen fibers similar in size to the collagen fibers of the living tendon, followed by making them into a tight bundle (not a simple twist string). In contrast, the top-down approach is the longitudinal fragmentation of a large bundle of uniaxially aligned collagen fibrils to allow infiltration of extrinsic cells.

Recently, the performance of decellularized tendons for ACL reconstruction has been evaluated *in vivo* [93, 94]. Although there are some challenges including unevenness of material qualities, residual sources of infection, and production costs, excellent mechanical features and collagen structures similar to living tissues are suitable for ACL reconstruction. The differences between collagen-based artificial tendons and decellularized tendons should be considered in biomaterial developments.

Acknowledgements

This work including the rheological experiments was supported by JSPS KAKENHI Grant Number 15 K01321.

Conflict of interest

The authors declare that they have no conflict of interest.

Author details

Shunji Yunoki[1]*, Eiji Kondo[2] and Kazunori Yasuda[3,4]

1 Biotechnology Group, Tokyo Metropolitan Industrial Technology Research Institute (TIRI), Tokyo, Japan

2 Department of Advanced Therapeutic Research for Sports Medicine, Hokkaido University Graduate School of Medicine, Sapporo, Japan

3 Department of Sports Medicine, Hokkaido University Graduate School of Medicine, Sapporo, Japan

4 Knee Research Center, Yagi Orthopaedic Hospital, Sapporo, Japan

*Address all correspondence to: yunokishuji530@gmail.com

References

[1] Yannas IV, Burke JF. Design of an artificial skin. I. Basic design principles. Journal of Biomedical Materials Research. 1980;**14**:65-81. DOI: 10.1002/jbm.820140108

[2] Yannas IV, Burke JF, Gordon PL, Huang C, Rubenstein RH. Design of an artificial skin. II. Control of chemical composition. Journal of Biomedical Materials Research. 1980;**14**:107-132. DOI: 10.1002/jbm.820140203

[3] Friess W. Collagen -biomaterial for drug delivery. European Journal of Pharmaceutics and Biopharmaceutics. 1998;**45**:113-136. DOI: 10.1016/s0939-6411(98)00017-4

[4] Lee CH, Singla A, Lee Y. Biomedical applications of collagen. International Journal of Pharmaceutics. 2001;**221**(1-2):1-22. DOI: 10.1016/s0378-5173(01)00691-3

[5] Liu X, Zheng C, Luo X, Wang X, Jiang H. Recent advances of collagen-based biomaterials: Multi-hierarchical structure, modification and biomedical applications. Materials Science & Engineering. C, Materials for Biological Applications. 2019;**99**:1509-1522. DOI: 10.1016/j.msec.2019.02.070

[6] Lin K, Zhang D, Macedo MH, Cui W, Sarmento B, Shen G. Advanced collagen-based biomaterials for regenerative biomedicine. Advanced Functional Materials. 2019;**29**:1804943. DOI: 10.1002/adfm.201804943

[7] Ruszczak Z. Effect of collagen matrices on dermal wound healing. Advanced Drug Delivery Reviews. 2003;**55**:1595-1611. DOI: 10.1016/j.addr.2003.08.003

[8] Ferreira AM, Gentile P, Chiono V, Ciardelli G. Collagen for bone tissue regeneration. Acta Biomaterialia. 2012;**8**(9):3191-3200. DOI: 10.1016/j.actbio.2012.06.014

[9] Responte DJ, Natoli RM, Athanasiou KA. Collagens of articular cartilage: Structure, function, and importance in tissue engineering. Critical Reviews in Biomedical Engineering. 2007;**35**(5):363-411. DOI: 10.1615/critrevbiomedeng.v35.i5.20

[10] Fratzl P. Collagen: Structure and mechanics, an introduction. In: Fratzl P, editor. Collagen Structure and Mechanics. Boston, MA: Springer; 2011. pp. 1-14. DOI: 10.1007/978-0-387-73906-9_1

[11] Silver FH, Freeman JW, Seehra GP. Collagen self-assembly and the development of tendon mechanical properties. Journal of Biomechanics. 2003;**36**(10):1529-1553. DOI: 10.1016/s0021-9290(03)00135-0

[12] Biewener AA. Tendons and ligaments: Structure, mechanical behavior and biological function. In: Fratzl P, editor. Collagen Structure and Mechanics. Boston, MA: Springer; 2011. pp. 269-284. DOI: 10.1007/978-0-387-73906-9_10

[13] Williams BR, Gelman RA, Poppke DC, Piez KA. Collagen fibril formation. Optimal in vitro conditions and preliminary kinetic results. The Journal of Biological Chemistry. 1978;**253**:6578-6585

[14] Harris JR, Reiber A. Influence of saline and pH on collagen type I fibrillogenesis in vitro: Fibril polymorphism and colloidal gold labelling. Micron. 2007;**38**:513-521. DOI: 10.1016/j.micron.2006.07.026

[15] Dewle A, Pathak N, Rakshasmare P, Srivastava A. Multifarious fabrication approaches of producing aligned collagen scaffolds for tissue engineering applications. ACS Biomaterials Science & Engineering. 2020;**6**:779-797. DOI: 10.1021/acsbiomaterials.9b01225

[16] No YJ, Castilho M, Ramaswamy Y, Zreiqat H. Role of biomaterials and controlled architecture on tendon/ligament repair and regeneration. Advanced Materials. 2020;**32**:e1904511. DOI: 10.1002/adma.201904511

[17] Ma C, Wang H, Chi Y, Wang Y, Jiang L, Xu N, et al. Preparation of oriented collagen fiber scaffolds and its application in bone tissue engineering. Applied Materials Today. 2021;**22**:100902. DOI: 10.1016/j.apmt.2020.100902

[18] Benjamin M, Ralphs JR. Tendons and ligaments -an overview. Histology and Histopathology. 1997;**12**:1135-1144. DOI: 10.14670/HH-12.1135

[19] Kew SJ, Gwynne JH, Enea D, Abu-Rub M, Pandit A, Zeugolis D, et al. Regeneration and repair of tendon and ligament tissue using collagen fibre biomaterials. Acta Biomaterialia. 2011;**7**:3237-3247. DOI: 10.1016/j.actbio.2011.06.002

[20] Fratzl P. Collagen: Hierarchical structure and viscoelastic properties of tendon. In: Shewry PR, Tatham AS, Bailey AJ, editors. Elastomeric Proteins: Structures, Biomechanical Properties, and Biological Roles. Vol. 2003. Cambridge, UK: Cambridge University Press; 2003. pp. 175-188

[21] Birch HL. Tendon matrix composition and turnover in relation to functional requirements. International Journal of Experimental Pathology. 2007;**88**:241-248. DOI: 10.1111/j.1365-2613.2007.00552.x

[22] Chandrashekar N, Mansouri H, Slauterbeck J, Hashemi J. Sex-based differences in the tensile properties of the human anterior cruciate ligament. Journal of Biomechanics. 2006;**39**:2943-2950. DOI: 10.1016/j.jbiomech.2005.10.031

[23] Alentorn-Geli E, Mendiguchía J, Samuelsson K, Musahl V, Karlsson J, Cugat R, et al. Prevention of anterior cruciate ligament injuries in sports. Part I: Systematic review of risk factors in male athletes. Knee Surgery, Sports Traumatology, Arthroscopy. 2014;**22**:3-15. DOI: 10.1007/s00167-013-2725-3

[24] Agel J, Arendt EA, Bershadsky B. Anterior cruciate ligament injury in National Collegiate Athletic Association basketball and soccer a 13-year review. The American Journal of Sports Medicine. 2005;**33**:524-531. DOI: 10.1177/0363546504269937

[25] Mall NA, Chalmers PN, Moric M, Tanaka MJ, Cole BJ, Bach BR Jr, et al. Incidence and trends of anterior cruciate ligament reconstruction in the United States. The American Journal of Sports Medicine. 2014;**42**:2363-2370. DOI: 10.1177/0363546514542796

[26] Levy BA, Dajani KA, Morgan JA, Shah JP, Dahm DL, Stuart MJ. Repair versus reconstruction of the fibular collateral ligament and posterolateral corner in the multiligament-injured knee. The American Journal of Sports Medicine. 2010;**38**:804-809. DOI: 10.1177/0363546509352459

[27] Ajrawat P, Dwyer T, Whelan D, Theodoropoulos J, Murnaghan L, Bhargava M, et al. A comparison of quadriceps tendon autograft with bone-patellar tendon-bone autograft and hamstring tendon autograft for primary anterior cruciate ligament reconstruction: A systematic review and

quantitative synthesis. Clinical Journal of Sport Medicine. 2021;**31**:392-399. DOI: 10.1097/JSM.0000000000000765 PMID: 31233432

[28] Pinczewski LA, Lyman J, Salmon LJ, Russell VJ, Roe J, Linklater J. A 10-year comparison of anterior cruciate ligament reconstructions with hamstring tendon and patellar tendon autograft: A controlled, prospective trial. The American Journal of Sports Medicine. 2007;**35**:564-574. DOI: 10.1177/0363546506296042

[29] Janssen RP, van der Wijk J, Fiedler A, Schmidt T, Sala HA, Scheffler SU. Remodelling of human hamstring autografts after anterior cruciate ligament reconstruction. Knee Surgery, Sports Traumatology, Arthroscopy. 2011;**19**:1299-1306. DOI: 10.1007/s00167-011-1419-y

[30] Tohyama H, Yasuda K, Uchida H. Is the increase in type III collagen of the patellar tendon graft after ligament reconstruction really caused by "ligamentization" of the graft? Knee Surgery, Sports Traumatology, Arthroscopy. 2006;**14**:1270-1277. DOI: 10.1007/s00167-006-0092-z

[31] Tohyama H, Yasuda K. Extrinsic cell infiltration and revascularization accelerate mechanical deterioration of the patellar tendon after fibroblast necrosis. Journal of Biomechanical Engineering. 2000;**122**:594-599. DOI: 10.1115/1.1319659

[32] Hardy A, Casabianca L, Andrieu K, Baverel L, Noailles T, Junior French Arthroscopy Society. Complications following harvesting of patellar tendon or hamstring tendon grafts for anterior cruciate ligament reconstruction: Systematic review of literature. Orthopaedics & Traumatology, Surgery & Research. 2017;**103**(8S):S245-S248. DOI: 10.1016/j.otsr.2017.09.002

[33] Murray MM. Current status and potential of primary ACL repair. Clinics in Sports Medicine. 2009;**28**:51-61. DOI: 10.1016/j.csm.2008.08.005

[34] Chen J, Xu J, Wang A, Zheng M. Scaffolds for tendon and ligament repair: Review of the efficacy of commercial products. Expert Review of Medical Devices. 2009;**6**(1):61-73. DOI: 10.1586/17434440.6.1.61

[35] Huang Z-M, Zhang Y-Z, Kotaki M, Ramakrishna S. A review on polymer nanofibers by electrospinning and their applications in nanocomposites. Composites Science and Technology. 2003;**63**:2223-2253. DOI: 10.1016/S0266-3538(03)00178-7

[36] Barnes CP, Sell SA, Boland ED, Simpson DG, Bowlin GL. Nanofiber technology: Designing the next generation of tissue engineering scaffolds. Advanced Drug Delivery Reviews. 2007;**59**:1413-1433. DOI: 10.1016/j.addr.2007.04.022

[37] Zhong S, Teo WE, Zhu X, Beuerman RW, Ramakrishna S, Yung LY. An aligned nanofibrous collagen scaffold by electrospinning and its effects on in vitro fibroblast culture. Journal of Biomedical Materials Research. Part A. 2006;**79**:456-463. DOI: 10.1002/jbm.a.30870

[38] Xu Y, Wu J, Wang H, Li H, Di N, Song L, et al. Fabrication of electrospun poly(L-lactide-co-ε-caprolactone)/collagen nanoyarn network as a novel, three-dimensional, macroporous, aligned scaffold for tendon tissue engineering. Tissue Engineering. Part C, Methods. 2013;**19**(12):925-936. DOI: 10.1089/ten.TEC.2012.0328

[39] Xu Y, Dong S, Zhou Q, Mo X, Song L, Hou T, et al. The effect of mechanical stimulation on the

maturation of TDSCs-poly(L-lactide-co-e-caprolactone)/collagen scaffold constructs for tendon tissue engineering. Biomaterials. 2014;**35**:2760-2772. DOI: 10.1016/j.biomaterials.2013.12.042

[40] Zeugolis DI, Khew ST, Yew ES, Ekaputra AK, Tong YW, Yung LY, et al. Electro-spinning of pure collagen nano-fibres -just an expensive way to make gelatin? Biomaterials. 2008;**29**:2293-2305. DOI: 10.1016/j.biomaterials.2008.02.009

[41] Matthews JA, Wnek GE, Simpson DG, Bowlin GL. Electrospinning of collagen nanofibers. Biomacromolecules. 2002;**3**:232-238. DOI: 10.1021/bm015533u

[42] Ciurzynska A, Lenart A. Freeze-drying-application in food processing and biotechnology—a review. Polish Journal of Food and Nutrition Sciences. 2011;**61**:165-171. DOI: 10.2478/v10222-011-0017-5

[43] Shukla S. Freeze drying process: A review. International Journal of Pharmaceutical Sciences and Research. 2011;**2**:3061-3068

[44] Wegst UG, Schecter M, Donius AE, Hunger PM. Biomaterials by freeze casting. Philosophical Transactions of the Royal Society A: Mathematical, Physical and Engineering Sciences. 1917;**2010**(368):2099-2121. DOI: 10.1098/rsta.2010.0014

[45] Schoof H, Bruns L, Fischer A, Heschel I, Rau G. Dendritic ice morphology in unidirectionally solidified collagen suspensions. Journal of Crystal Growth. 2000;**209**:122-129. DOI: 10.1016/S0022-0248(99)00519-9

[46] Schoof H, Apel J, Heschel I, Rau G. Control of pore structure and size in freeze-dried collagen sponges. Journal of Biomedical Materials Research Part B: Applied Biomaterials. 2001;**58**:352-357. DOI: 10.1002/jbm.1028

[47] Zhang H, Cooper AI. Aligned porous structures by directional freezing. Advanced Materials. 2007;**19**:1529-1533. DOI: 10.1002/adma.200700154

[48] Pot MW, Faraj KA, Adawy A, van Enckevort WJ, van Moerkerk HT, Vlieg E, et al. Versatile wedge-based system for the construction of unidirectional collagen scaffolds by directional freezing: Practical and theoretical considerations. ACS Applied Materials & Interfaces. 2015;**7**:8495-8505. DOI: 10.1021/acsami.5b00169

[49] Zheng Z, Ran J, Chen W, Hu Y, Zhu T, Chen X, et al. Alignment of collagen fiber in knitted silk scaffold for functional massive rotator cuff repair. Acta Biomaterialia. 2017;**51**:317-329. DOI: 10.1016/j.actbio.2017.01.041

[50] Lowe CJ, Reucroft IM, Grota MC, Shreiber DI. Production of highly aligned collagen scaffolds by freeze-drying of self-assembled, fibrillar collagen gels. ACS Biomaterials Science & Engineering. 2016;**2**:643-651. DOI: 10.1021/acsbiomaterials.6b00036

[51] Torbet J, Ronzière MC. Magnetic alignment of collagen during self-assembly. The Biochemical Journal. 1984;**219**(3):1057-0159. DOI: 10.1042/bj2191057

[52] Dickinson RB, Guido S, Tranquillo RT. Biased cell migration of fibroblasts exhibiting contact guidance in oriented collagen gels. Annals of Biomedical Engineering. 1994;**22**: 342-356. DOI: 10.1007/BF02368241

[53] Chen S, Hirota N, Okuda M, Takeguchi M, Kobayashi H, Hanagata N, et al. Microstructures and rheological properties of tilapia fish-scale

collagen hydrogels with aligned fibrils fabricated under magnetic fields. Acta Biomaterialia. 2011;7:644-652. DOI: 10.1016/j.actbio.2010.09.014

[54] Torbet J, Malbouyres M, Builles N, Justin V, Roulet M, Damour O, et al. Orthogonal scaffold of magnetically aligned collagen lamellae for corneal stroma reconstruction. Biomaterials. 2007;**28**(29):4268-4276. DOI: 10.1016/j.biomaterials.2007.05.024

[55] Sharma S, Panitch A, Neu CP. Incorporation of an aggrecan mimic prevents proteolytic degradation of anisotropic cartilage analogs. Acta Biomaterialia. 2013;**9**:4618-4625. DOI: 10.1016/j.actbio.2012.08.041

[56] Novak T, Voytik-Harbin SL, Neu CP. Cell encapsulation in a magnetically aligned collagen-GAG copolymer microenvironment. Acta Biomaterialia. 2015;**11**:274-282. DOI: 10.1016/j.actbio.2014.09.031

[57] Antman-Passig M, Shefi O. Remote magnetic orientation of 3D collagen hydrogels for directed neuronal regeneration. Nano Letters. 2016;**16**(4):2567-2573. DOI: 10.1021/acs.nanolett.6b00131

[58] Sharma A, DiVito MD, Shore DE, Block AD, Pollock K, Solheid P, et al. Alignment of collagen matrices using magnetic nanowires and magnetic barcode readout using first order reversal curves (FORC). Journal of Magnetism and Magnetic Materials. 2018;**459**:176-181. DOI: 10.1016/j.jmmm.2017.11.035

[59] Taufalele PV, VanderBurgh JA, Muñoz A, Zanotelli MR, Reinhart-King CA. Fiber alignment drives changes in architectural and mechanical features in collagen matrices. PLoS One. 2019;**14**:e0216537. DOI: 10.1371/journal.pone.0216537

[60] Shi Y, Li Y, Coradin T. Magnetically-oriented type I collagen-SiO_2@Fe_3O_4 rods composite hydrogels tuning skin cell growth. Colloids and Surfaces. B, Biointerfaces. 2020;**185**:110597. DOI: 10.1016/j.colsurfb.2019.110597

[61] Cheng X, Gurkan UA, Dehen CJ, Tate MP, Hillhouse HW, Simpson GJ, et al. An electrochemical fabrication process for the assembly of anisotropically oriented collagen bundles. Biomaterials. 2008;**29**(22):3278-3288. DOI: 10.1016/j.biomaterials.2008.04.028

[62] Younesi M, Islam A, Kishore V, Anderson JM, Akkus O. Tenogenic induction of human MSCs by anisotropically aligned collagen biotextiles. Advanced Functional Materials. 2014;**24**:5762-5770. DOI: 10.1002/adfm.201400828

[63] Gurkan UA, Cheng X, Kishore V, Uquillas JA, Akkus O. Comparison of morphology, orientation, and migration of tendon derived fibroblasts and bone marrow stromal cells on electrochemically aligned collagen constructs. Journal of Biomedical Materials Research. Part A. 2010;**94**:1070-1079. DOI: 10.1002/jbm.a.32783

[64] Abu-Rub MT, Billiar KL, Van Es MH, Knight A, Rodriguez BJ, Zeugolis DI, et al. Nano-textured self-assembled aligned collagen hydrogels promote directional neurite guidance and overcome inhibition by myelin associated glycoprotein. Soft Matter. 2011;**7**:2770-2781. DOI: 10.1039/C0SM01062F

[65] Kishore V, Bullock W, Sun X, Van Dyke WS, Akkus O. Tenogenic differentiation of human MSCs induced by the topography of electrochemically aligned collagen threads. Biomaterials. 2012;**33**:2137-2144. DOI: 10.1016/j.biomaterials.2011.11.066

[66] Chen Z, Liu X, You J, Song Y, Tomaskovic-Crook E, Sutton G, et al. Biomimetic corneal stroma using electro-compacted collagen. Acta Biomaterialia. 2020;**113**:360-371. DOI: 10.1016/j.actbio.2020.07.004

[67] Learn GD, McClellan PE, Knapik DM, Cumsky JL, Webster-Wood V, Anderson JM, et al. Woven collagen biotextiles enable mechanically functional rotator cuff tendon regeneration during repair of segmental tendon defects in vivo. Journal of Biomedical Materials Research. Part B, Applied Biomaterials. 2019;**107**:1864-1876. DOI: 10.1002/jbm.b.34279

[68] Kato YP, Christiansen DL, Hahn RA, Shieh SJ, Goldstein JD, Silver FH. Mechanical properties of collagen fibres: A comparison of reconstituted and rat tail tendon fibres. Biomaterials. 1989;**10**:38-42. DOI: 10.1016/0142-9612(89)90007-0

[69] Kew SJ, Gwynne JH, Enea D, Brookes R, Rushton N, Best SM, et al. Synthetic collagen fascicles for the regeneration of tendon tissue. Acta Biomaterialia. 2012;**8**:3723-3731. DOI: 10.1016/j.actbio.2012.06.018

[70] Dunn MG, Avasarala PN, Zawadsky JP. Optimization of extruded collagen fibers for ACL reconstruction. Journal of Biomedical Materials Research. 1993;**27**:1545-1552. DOI: 10.1002/jbm.820271211

[71] Cavallaro JF, Kemp PD, Kraus KH. Collagen fabrics as biomaterials. Biotechnology and Bioengineering. 1994;**43**(8):781-791. DOI: 10.1002/bit.260430813

[72] Siriwardane ML, DeRosa K, Collins G, Pfister BJ. Controlled formation of cross-linked collagen fibers for neural tissue engineering applications. Biofabrication. 2014;**6**:015012. DOI: 10.1088/1758-5082/6/1/015012

[73] Zeugolis DI, Paul RG, Attenburrow G. Post-self-assembly experimentation on extruded collagen fibres for tissue engineering applications. Acta Biomaterialia. 2008;**4**:1646-1656. DOI: 10.1016/j.actbio.2008.05.015

[74] Pins GD, Christiansen DL, Patel R, Silver FH. Self-assembly of collagen fibers. Influence of fibrillar alignment and decorin on mechanical properties. Biophysical Journal. 1997;**73**:2164-2172. DOI: 10.1016/S0006-3495(97)78247-X

[75] Nerger BA, Brun PT, Nelson CM. Microextrusion printing cell-laden networks of type I collagen with patterned fiber alignment and geometry. Soft Matter. 2019;**15**:5728-5738. DOI: 10.1039/c8sm02605j

[76] Lai ES, Anderson CM, Fuller GG. Designing a tubular matrix of oriented collagen fibrils for tissue engineering. Acta Biomaterialia. 2011;**7**:2448-2456. DOI: 10.1016/j.actbio.2011.03.012

[77] Caves JM, Kumar VA, Wen J, Cui W, Martinez A, Apkarian R, et al. Fibrillogenesis in continuously spun synthetic collagen fiber. Journal of Biomedical Materials Research. Part B, Applied Biomaterials. 2010;**93**:24-38. DOI: 10.1002/jbm.b.31555

[78] Malladi S, Miranda-Nieves D, Leng L, Grainger SJ, Tarabanis C, Nesmith AP, et al. Continuous formation of ultrathin, strong collagen sheets with tunable anisotropy and compaction. ACS Biomaterials Science & Engineering. 2020;**6**:4236-4246. DOI: 10.1021/acsbiomaterials.0c00321

[79] Lai ES, Huang NF, Cooke JP, Fuller GG. Aligned nanofibrillar collagen regulates endothelial organization and migration. Regenerative Medicine. 2012;**7**:649-661. DOI: 10.2217/rme.12.48

[80] Ziolko FJ. Method of Making a Tubular Collagen Casing. Somerville,

NJ, USA: Devro Inc.; 1979. Patent No: US4138503.

[81] Hoogenkamp HR, Bakker GJ, Wolf L, Suurs P, Dunnewind B, Barbut S, et al. Directing collagen fibers using counter-rotating cone extrusion. Acta Biomaterialia. 2015;**12**:113-121. DOI: 10.1016/j.actbio.2014.10.012

[82] Yang S, Shi X, Li X, Wang J, Wang Y, Luo Y. Oriented collagen fiber membranes formed through counter-rotating extrusion and their application in tendon regeneration. Biomaterials. 2019;**207**:61-75. DOI: 10.1016/j.biomaterials.2019.03.041

[83] Yunoki S, Sugimoto K, Ohyabu Y, Ida H, Hiraoka Y. Accurate and precise viscosity measurements of gelatin solutions using a rotational rheometer. Food Science and Technology Research. 2019;**25**:217-226. DOI: 10.3136/fstr.25.217

[84] Saeidi N, Sander EA, Ruberti JW. Dynamic shear-influenced collagen self-assembly. Biomaterials. 2009;**30**:6581-6592. DOI: 10.1016/j.biomaterials.2009.07.070

[85] Saeidi N, Sander EA, Zareian R, Ruberti JW. Production of highly aligned collagen lamellae by combining shear force and thin film confinement. Acta Biomaterialia. 2011;7:2437-2447. DOI: 10.1016/j.actbio.2011.02.038

[86] Lanfer B, Freudenberg U, Zimmermann R, Stamov D, Körber V, Werner C. Aligned fibrillar collagen matrices obtained by shear flow deposition. Biomaterials. 2008;**29**(28): 3888-3895. DOI: 10.1016/j.biomaterials.2008.06.016

[87] Lanfer B, Seib FP, Freudenberg U, Stamov D, Bley T, Bornhäuser M, et al. The growth and differentiation of mesenchymal stem and progenitor cells cultured on aligned collagen matrices. Biomaterials. 2009;**30**:5950-5958. DOI: 10.1016/j.biomaterials.2009.07.039

[88] Lanfer B, Hermann A, Kirsch M, Freudenberg U, Reuner U, Werner C, et al. Directed growth of adult human white matter stem cell-derived neurons on aligned fibrillar collagen. Tissue Engineering. Part A. 2010;**16**(4):1103-1113. DOI: 10.1089/ten.TEA.2009.0282

[89] Giraud-Guille MM, Besseau L, Martin R. Liquid crystalline assemblies of collagen in bone and in vitro systems. Journal of Biomechanics. 2003;**36**:1571-1579. DOI: 10.1016/s0021-9290(03)00134-9

[90] Paten JA, Siadat SM, Susilo ME, Ismail EN, Stoner JL, Rothstein JP, et al. Flow-induced crystallization of collagen: A potentially critical mechanism in early tissue formation. ACS Nano. 2016;**10**:5027-5040. DOI: 10.1021/acsnano.5b07756

[91] Yunoki S, Hatayama H, Ebisawa M, Kondo E, Yasuda K. A novel fabrication method to create a thick collagen bundle composed of uniaxially aligned fibrils: An essential technology for the development of artificial tendon/ligament matrices. Journal of Biomedical Materials Research. Part A. 2015;**103**:3054-3065. DOI: 10.1002/jbm.a.35440

[92] Yunoki S, Hatayama H, Ebisawa M, Kondo E, Yasuda K. A novel method for continuous formation of cord-like collagen gels to fabricate durable fibers in which collagen fibrils are longitudinally aligned. Journal of Biomedical Materials Research. Part B, Applied Biomaterials. 2019;**107**:1011-1023. DOI: 10.1002/jbm.b.34194

[93] Schulze-Tanzil G, Al-Sadi O, Ertel W, Lohan A. Decellularized tendon

extracellular matrix-a valuable approach for tendon reconstruction? Cell. 2012;**1**:1010-1028. DOI: 10.3390/cells1041010

[94] Li Y, Zhu T, Wang L, Jiang J, Xie G, Huangfu X, et al. Tissue-engineered decellularized allografts for anterior cruciate ligament reconstruction. ACS Biomaterials Science & Engineering. 2020;**6**:5700-5710. DOI: 10.1021/acsbiomaterials.0c00269